THE 20-MINUTE BODY

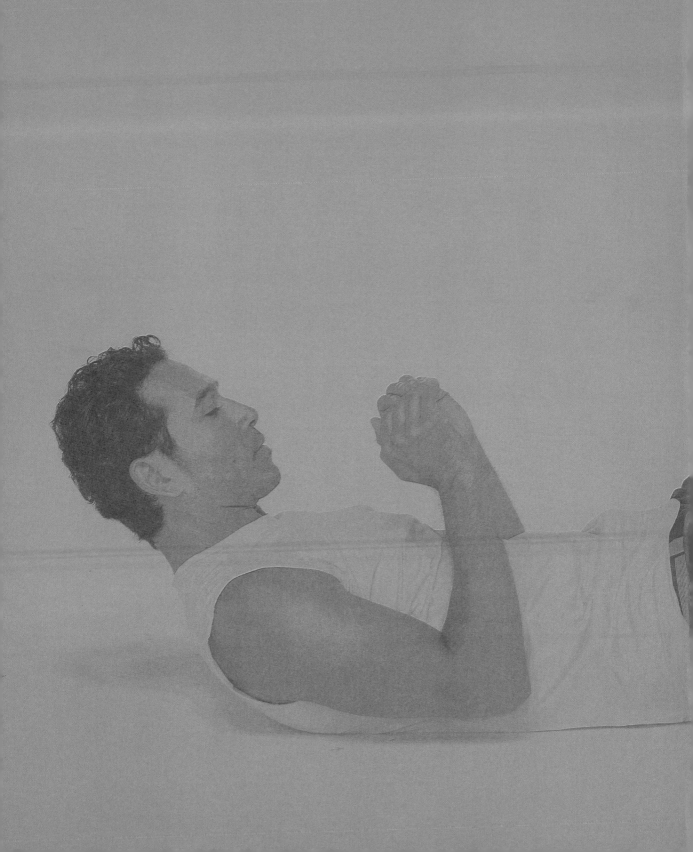

THE *THE* 20-MINUTE BODY

20 Minutes, 20 Days, 20 Inches

BRETT HOEBEL

HARPER WAVE

An Imprint of HarperCollinsPublishers

THE 20-MINUTE BODY. Copyright © 2015 by Brett Hoebel. All rights reserved. Printed in the United States of America. No part of this book may be used or reproduced in any manner whatsoever without written permission except in the case of brief quotations embodied in critical articles and reviews. For information, address HarperCollins Publishers, 195 Broadway, New York, NY 10007.

Image Credits: page 10 ©Ammentorp Photography/Shutterstock, Inc.; page 18 © Iaroslav Neliubov/Shutterstock, Inc.; page 21 ©Yanas/Shutterstock, Inc.; page 40 © Robyn Mackenzie/Shutterstock, Inc.; page 60 © rickyd/Shutterstock, Inc.; page 63 © symbiot/Shutterstock, Inc.; page 70 © Juriah Mosin/Shutterstock, Inc.; page 102 © Nadezhda Kulikova/Shutterstock, Inc.; page 113–115: tongs, sheers, knives, cutting board, microplane ©Katsiaryna Pleshakova/Shutterstock, Inc.; immersion blender, coffee grinder ©ayax/Shutterstock, Inc.; food processor © losw/Shutterstock, Inc,; water bottle © Dinko Bence/Shutterstock, Inc.; food scale © Krylovochka/Shutterstock, Inc.; page 118 © PKpix/Shutterstock, Inc.; page 224© Alis Leonte/Shutterstock, Inc.

HarperCollins books may be purchased for educational, business, or sales promotional use. For information, please e-mail the Special Markets Department at SPsales@harpercollins.com.

FIRST EDITION

Designed by Leah Carlson-Stanisic

Photography by Todd Vitti unless otherwise noted

Library of Congress Cataloging-in-Publication Data

Hoebel, Brett.

The 20-minute body : 20 minutes, 20 days, 20 inches / Brett Hoebel.

pages cm

ISBN 978-0-06-231678-3 (hardback)

1. Reducing exercises. 2. Reducing diets. 3. Physical fitness. 4. Weight loss. I. Title.

RA781.6.H64 2015

613.7—dc23

2014044383

14 15 16 17 18 OV/QG 10 9 8 7 6 5 4 3 2 1

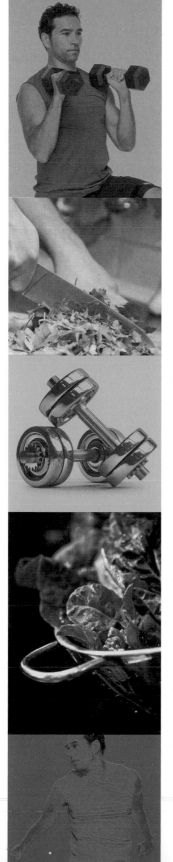

CONTENTS

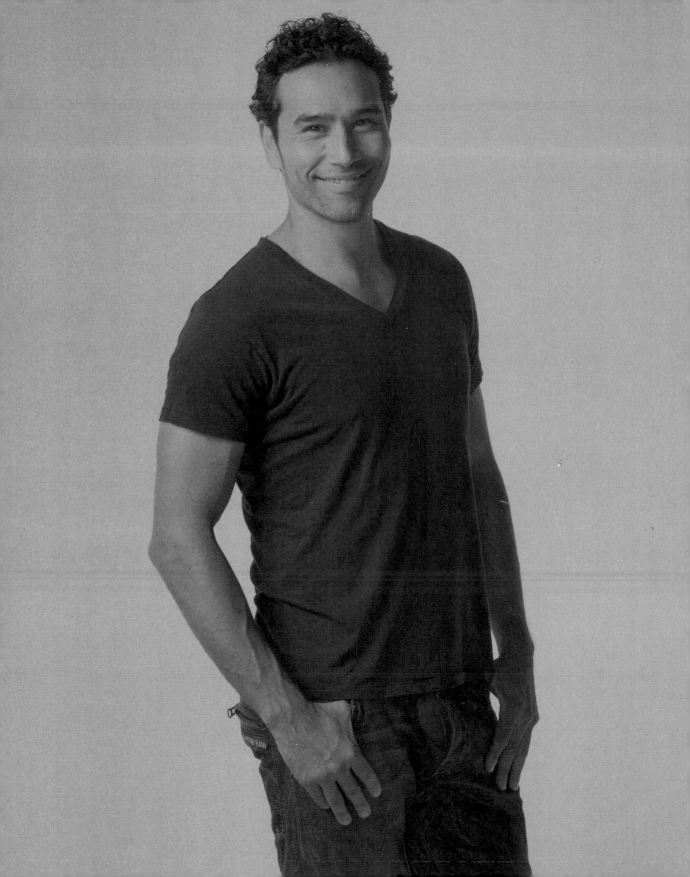

INTRODUCTION

My name is Brett Hoebel and I'm a fitness trainer, capoeira practitioner, and master motivator. I believe that results are not given, but earned, which is probably why those who have trained with me call me the "Dues Collector." You might know me from my work as a trainer on *The Biggest Loser* Season 11 or from one of my fitness DVDs. Or you may not know me at all—but if you've picked up this book, we're about to get to know each other very well!

Over the next 20 days, I will help you get stronger, leaner, and healthier. Through calculated, high-efficiency doses of exercise, no-fuss meal planning, and a careful recalibration of your mental approach to physical transformation, you'll achieve things that you never thought possible. This book is the product of more than ten years of experience training clients just like you—busy but health-minded individuals looking for ways to lose weight or stay fit without spending hours in the gym or starving themselves at every meal.

Today is your first step in a life-changing journey. So I think it's only fair that before we begin, I share a little bit about my own journey, too.

THE BEGINNING

I know what it feels like to be uncomfortable and ashamed of your body. As a teenager, I was overweight. In elementary school I had been diagnosed with a wheat allergy and I was hyperactive—double threat for a kid, right? When you have those labels, you have to contend with a lot of things that most "normal" kids don't. One of those things was my diet. Every time I'd walk into the lunchroom at school, there was a huge spread of food that was off-limits for me. While my friends were serving themselves pizza and mac 'n' cheese, I was reaching for chicken and vegetables. You ever try to choke down bland chicken while someone else is noshing on pizza? It's pretty much the worst kind of torture imaginable, especially in elementary school.

Plus, my tray looked different from everyone else's and just like any kid, I wanted to fit in. So I devised a system where I'd slyly stand behind friends in line and convince them to order the foods I wanted, and then I'd swap with them, or sometimes they'd just offer me the foods I knew I shouldn't have. Of course, I felt I was very clever. I didn't have to suffer the indignity of ridicule, nor did I have to suffer the lunchroom's most tasteless offerings.

Things got out of control from there. I had gained a lot of weight as a result of my cafeteria antics and this presented yet another hurdle to overcome when our family moved from New Jersey to California and I immediately stood out . . . again. I was picked last in sports. I was bullied. Eventually, because I had become too big, my gymnastics coach had to dismiss me from his program, even though I had been told I had a lot of potential. My weight was costing me a lot.

Feeling depressed and rejected, I latched on to any excuse I could think of not to go to school. So I would ditch, stay home, and eat all day and watch Bruce Lee movies. I liked eating, sure, but I was *enthralled* with Bruce Lee. I'd practice his moves in front of the TV, occasionally with a spoon in hand or crumbs on my shirt.

It just so happened that there was a martial arts studio along our route to school. My mom noticed how I'd rubberneck and drag my feet as we passed by each day and one day, she suggested that we go in. Inside, I noticed a kid about my age setting up for a board break. *This should be interesting.* I remember thinking that there was no way that this kid was up to it—he was heavy and not very athletic. Then, *crack.* Heavy kid 1, boards 0.

I was in. I signed up and before long, I was the one going up against half-inch boards and tussling with classmates in contact drills. During one of my first sparring matches, I was pitted against that same heavy kid I saw on my first visit. Wouldn't you know it? He destroyed me. And I loved it.

That karate school had given me my mojo back. So what did I do? Like any kid who had been tormented by his peers, I went back to campus and immediately got into two fights against kids who had been giving me a hard time. I wasn't going to take it anymore. I was back.

Except that shortly thereafter we moved back to New Jersey. In junior high it seemed to be an unwritten rule that you are *not* allowed to be friends with fat kids. It was terrible. I resorted to my old ways and I fell into a deeper depression.

I kept overeating, only now, a bit older, I started to become more aware of how detrimental it was. I knew that I shouldn't be doing it—and one look in the mirror was enough to remind me of that fact. Around this time, my mom, who had her own issues with weight, began to take more of an interest in my health, gently suggesting that I refrain from a second helping at dinner or that maybe I should skip dessert.

It got worse later. My mom organized her pantry with the detail of a librarian. If something was out of place or missing, she knew instantly. Amid a multi-tiered array of boxes and cans, she would know at a glance if a box of pasta or some cookies had been taken or even tampered with. This put me at another crossroads. What do I do when she shoots down my quest for satiety? The answer is not one I'm proud of.

One day, I found myself hiding on the floor of my bedroom closet, scarfing down junk food, pausing between bites to listen for approaching footsteps. Then it hit me. *What am I doing?* Well, among other things, I was increasing the odds that I would never kiss a girl. My obsession with food was putting normal adolescent milestones out of reach and it had to stop.

There, among my shoes and dirty clothes, I determined that I was going to reverse course and that my promises—both to myself and to others—were sacred. I couldn't go back on my word anymore. I was suddenly hyperaware that if I said I was going to do something—in this first case, lose some weight—then I had to do it.

FITNESS FROM WITHIN

And that brings us back to you. You no doubt picked up this book to help you increase your fitness levels, to help you dramatically improve your look and your performance levels. The reason I'm sharing the humiliation of my teenage years is to convey one point about your journey: the level of change that you can expect is a direct result of your accountability to your word. Getting in shape is hard, and staying that way is a daily decision and a lifelong commitment.

What tells you not to reach for that doughnut in the morning? What drags you out of bed to get in your workout when all you want to do is catch that extra 20 minutes of sleep? What compels you to prep veggies for a snack instead of grabbing a handful of chips? These decisions aren't the result of buying a magic gym membership or a fancy training gimmick. They are the result of *fitness from within*.

It's this inner drive that takes you deeper than the how-to of getting fit. It's about *why*. For me, it was a deep desire to be accepted, to just feel normal. Fatigued from a life chock-full of soul-rending rejection and exclusion, I decided that it was time for me to retake control of my body. Amid all of childhood's other uncertainties, this seemed more within my control.

This reason is different for every person but it needs to be sought out, identified, and converted into action. You have to get emotionally connected to your physical well-being. The workouts and the food, both of which I'm going to help you get straight over the next 20 days, are maybe 50 percent of this battle. The other half of it is finding your "why."

It could be that you want to feel beautiful for your spouse. Maybe you want to be able to keep up with your kids, return to your favorite sport, reduce your risk of disease, or just roll the clock back a few years. Whatever it is, knowing your "why" is crucial to following through. I assure you that if you can answer that question for yourself, the rest of what I have in store for you will yield much better results, and be more enjoyable.

What I will ask you to do in this program will seem difficult. There'll be times when you want to give up. But I promise you that none of it is impossible, and you will be better equipped to deal with the mental weakness that causes most people to fail if you spend a little time thinking about your "why," finding your own fitness from within.

THREE DISCIPLINES, 20 MINUTES, 20 INCHES, 20 DAYS

People think that training hard is the main component of any fitness program. Well, if getting fit were that easy, the gym would be filled with a bunch of skinny people. But it's not. It's full of people just like you— people who struggle with busy schedules, family obligations, work, school, and commutes and who may not have hours to spend in the gym or the wherewithal to prepare healthy meals after a long day. Fitness starts from within and it needs to follow you into the kitchen and every other aspect of your life. My program calls for you to discipline yourself in three areas—not just one. By dedicating just 20 minutes to these things throughout your day, you will be well on your way to dropping 20 inches from all over your body in 20 days. You'll lose more after that, for sure, but you will be amazed at what you do in your first 20.

The workouts in this book aren't based on the usual array of moderate cardio and dumbbell sets. No, this program is based on high-intensity cardio and strength training that conditions your body to be a lean, calorie-scorching machine in only a small fraction of the time that most workouts take. And the same applies to the kitchen. People think that meal planning and preparation are a time investment that they are ill equipped to pay into. But with a few kitchen-tested shortcuts and quick-prep secrets, I will help you remove that excuse as well.

• **20-MINUTE WORKOUTS:** Many people think that in order to get strong, lean muscles, they have to work out *longer*. They commit to these marathon treadmill sessions and routinely put in hours of steady-state cardio per week. Even those who train with weights get it wrong by training the same body parts every time, over-individualizing (i.e., training only biceps or focusing on shoulders), spending too much time with the same weights, or just using the wrong kinds of exercises. In both cases, there are greater results to be had by simply increasing the focus and intensity of the work. By shortening your workouts into all-out 20-minute sessions, you activate your fat-fighting machinery. And here's the thing: it *stays* activated for 1–2 days. I'll show you how (and why) a shorter time commitment each day can change your body dramatically and in far less time than traditional workouts.

• **20-MINUTE NUTRITION:** As I found out when I was younger, nutrition can make or break your get-lean efforts. What they say is true: no matter how hard you work out, you can never out-train a bad diet. But eating the right foods can seem daunting. Not everyone has the kitchen skills—or the hours of prep time—of a TV chef. I travel a lot. I know this. I know that getting a meal with protein, veggies, and a healthy carb takes careful planning and prep work. But as I've learned, there are a few easy ways—time management hacks, if you will—that can help you put together healthy, savory, minimalist meals that will speed your fat loss while providing plenty of energy for your workouts. You'll be amazed at what you can do with just a few ingredients, a dollop of food prep savvy, and 20 minutes of kitchen time. Once you have these recipes down, you'll never be at a loss for how to eat healthy again. And you'll finally have your eyes opened to just how tasty healthy eating can be!

• **20-MINUTE MINDSET:** That's right. Training your brain is just as important as training your body. You can condition your gray matter to do just about anything if you invest the time. This often-overlooked aspect of physique-building is crucial to setting, sticking to, and achieving your goals in the gym, in the kitchen, and, I would argue, in life. I'll let you in on some of the brain-training I do that can help steel your focus and speed your progress. This time is vital for reinforcing your "why," and it is the cornerstone of my *fitness from within* philosophy and can be done in as little as *20 minutes per week.* As my own experience taught me, long-lasting results hinge on your commitment to this cerebral but success-ensuring step.

YELLOW, ORANGE, BLUE

As I stated up front, I am a practitioner of the Afro-Brazilian art of capoeira ("kap-way-rah"), which combines elements of dance with martial arts. One attractive element of this discipline for me has always been the focus on progression. As you move up and learn new skills, you "graduate" to different-color cords (yellow, orange, and blue). But no matter your skill level at the beginning, everyone starts at white. Level playing field. That system inspired me to create a similar color system for the *20-Minute Body.*

Here, everyone starts at yellow. At the yellow level, which lasts 20 days, you learn how to perform effective yet fundamental movements that you can build on, you'll get some painless but healthy food upgrades in the kitchen, and your mindset training will be simple. And this initiation period will still be a very fruitful time for fat loss, I promise you. It will be a change but not the kind of cold-water shock that would impel you set this book on the shelf to collect dust like so many others. But as you build strength and discipline, your body will want—no, *need*—additional challenges to continue changing. The orange level, another 20-day evolution, steps it up in the exercise department, cleans up foods that you're already eating, and helps you get more practiced with your mindset exercises. The blue level continues that trend for another 20 days, taking things up a notch with higher-octane moves and routines. At this point, more than 40 days in, you'll also be seeing crazy results both in the mirror and in your performance.

And when you're done with the blue level, you can repeat the blue workouts, or take your newfound strength and stamina back to yellow or orange and crush your previous best results to provide a new jolt of confidence! Of course, since blue represents the pinnacle of cleaner eating, you'll want to stay as close to that as possible, but your workout options are literally endless.

This built-in progression allows you to achieve results at a rapid but sustainable pace while also keeping you from getting discouraged or injured. The bonus? You have not just 20, but 60 days of fat-shedding wisdom. And you will never get bored, because I'm constantly changing things up on you. I will make you move differently, go faster, rest less, and eat cleaner. You will always face a new challenge that keeps you interested and inspired as you watch the pounds and inches drop away.

I was a heavy kid with a lot of things working against me. I hid behind food until I hid under dozens of pounds of unwanted body fat. I allowed impulsive, emotional eating to overtake me to the point of depression and poor health. I stopped making time for things that made me happy. For so long, I let other people dictate my own personal worth. I made light of my lack of discipline, turning eating into a sport.

All facades. All excuses. Any of this sound familiar?

I overcame all of that. For good. And so can you. With this book, I'm going to help you drop the act and tear down the barriers that are standing between you and a body you can be proud of—one whose outer strength is surpassed only by that which lies within.

You ready to lose 20 inches in 20 days? Then it's time to turn the page—both literally and figuratively—and get started.

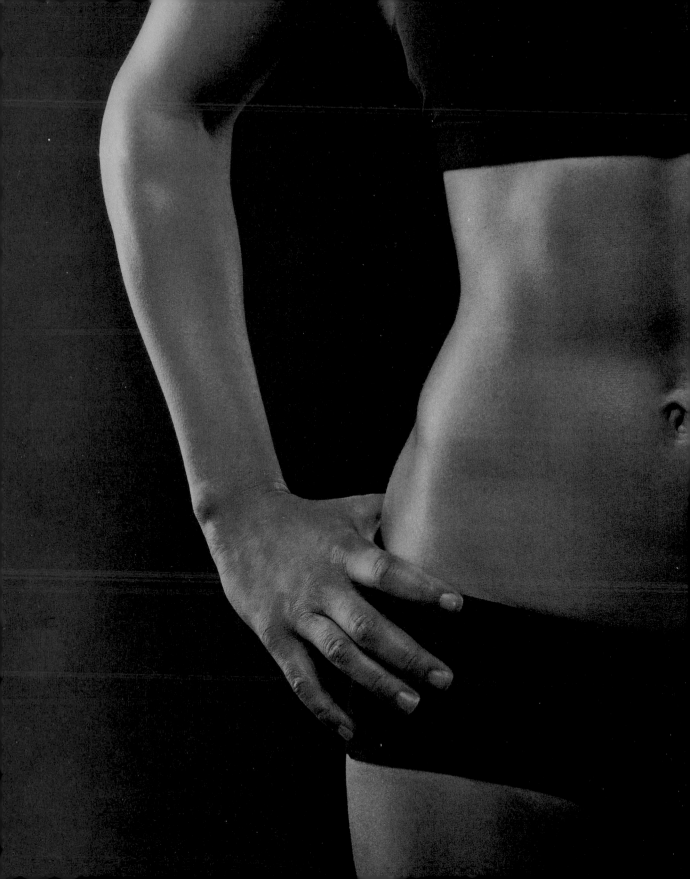

ONE

Hidden Muscle

THE SECRET TO A FAST METABOLISM, FAST WEIGHT LOSS,
AND A BETTER LEVEL OF FITNESS

EVERYWHERE I TRAVEL, it seems that people approach me with the same diet and training conundrums: serial missteps that have produced little in the way of lasting body change and, in some cases, even create frustrating setbacks. They stem from bad habits, bad information, or some combination of both. But as I tell these people, bad habits can be unlearned and bad info can be replaced by proven science. If your goal is to redefine your body, you first have to redefine your understanding of how it works.

When people decide that it's time to lose a few pounds, the focus is generally on getting rid of fat, not gaining muscle. And with a fat-first focus on losing weight, plateaus come quickly and often. Almost by instinct, people put themselves through unnecessary deprivation—eliminating carbs or fat, or bringing calorie levels down to dangerously low levels—in an attempt to starve out or kill fat cells (see the table on page 12). This approach is a pandemic that has swallowed up so much of our population, but I think a cure is within reach.

BODY FAT LEVELS IN ADULTS

Description	Women	Men
MINIMUM LEVEL	10–13%	2–5%
ATHLETES	14–20%	6–13%
FIT PEOPLE	21–24%	14–17%
AVERAGE	25–31%	18–24%
OBESE	32%+	25%+

You can get your body fat percentage taken by a professional to see where you fall on this scale.

IT'S NOT ABOUT FAT, IT'S ABOUT MUSCLE

Forget about losing fat. The key to everything is muscle—you have to train it, gain it, and maintain it in order to keep your body *metabolic*. Proportionally speaking, the more lean muscle your body has, the more calories your body will burn at rest. That bears repeating: *the more lean muscle your body has, the more calories your body will burn at rest.* That doesn't mean that you need to have the biceps of a bodybuilder to see results; you can optimize your existing muscle to make it work for you around the clock. Understanding the concept of *metabolic muscle* is perhaps the greatest, yet most tragically underused asset in our quest to become fitter. *Metabolic muscle* is the secret to fast metabolism.

So what is metabolic muscle? Simply put, it's muscle that has become highly efficient at using energy (read: burning fat and calories) through proper training and nutrition. Metabolic muscle motivates your body to burn more fat. It is something that you can work toward, regardless of how much muscle you were born with and regardless of your skill level, and this fact should encourage and empower you.

THE MAGIC OF METABOLIC MUSCLE

Picture a sprinter and a marathon runner. Both athletes train hard but the sprinter, whose training focuses on high-intensity work, has great muscle definition and carries a very low percentage of body fat. The marathoner, on the other hand, tends to have smaller muscles and may even carry a bit more fat.

Here's why that comparison matters: focusing on attacking those large muscle groups with intense, interval-based activity will do more for your body composition than the all-day cardio sessions that people too often lean on for weight loss. I am going to teach you to "sprint" your way to a new body, so to speak. When you turn up the heat on your training, you turn up the demand on these metabolic muscles—just like a sprinter.

And here's the best part: these muscles don't just call it a day when the workout is over. Turning up the intensity on your workouts takes advantage of a biological phenomenon known as "excess post-exercise oxygen consumption," or EPOC. You may have heard this referred to elsewhere as the "afterburn." Regardless of what you call it, this is something that benefits you greatly. It accounts for the amount of energy that your body has to burn in the 24–48 hours after the conclusion of a workout (depending on intensity and duration) to recover and return to a normal, resting state. Any kind of training can produce this effect, but it is maximized through exercise that zeroes in on this metabolic muscle—the kind of exercise that you'll be doing for the next 20 days.

So while you're sitting at the kitchen table helping your kids with homework, paying your bills online, or catching up on your DVR'd episodes of *The Good Wife*, your body is still torching calories and fat. How's that for return on investment?

Training for metabolic muscle makes so much sense for so many reasons. It is absolutely the results-boosting, time-saving, body-redefining upgrade that you've been looking for. All of those days, months, and years of unproductive training methods that have brought you to this point will be a distant memory after the next 20 days.

WORK OUT FOR MINUTES, NOT HOURS

What sounds better to you? Workouts where your fat-burning stops when you stop? Or workouts that silently shape you into a metabolic machine for hours and days after you leave the gym?

Long, steady-state cardio, where you're running (or biking) at the same pace for extended periods of time, doesn't offer much in the way of after-burn. Your energy use pretty much stops when you stop moving (or very shortly after). It is true that this type of cardio generally burns a lot of calories *during* a workout but that's where the benefits end. Hey, that's great if you have nothing but time (and energy) to burn but most of us have work to do, families to support, classes to sit through, commutes to endure.

Need further incentive to train for metabolic muscle? A 1994 study in the journal *Metabolism*[1] found that an interval-training group lost three times more subcutaneous fat (the type of fat found just beneath your skin) than an endurance training group. Hard bouts of exercise with built-in periods of recovery were found to be a better way to burn fat. And the research has only continued to mount since then. *Who knew?* This means that training with a more metabolic slant can help you preferentially burn the fat just beneath your skin, the type that obscures the muscular detail that most of us would like to reveal.

I don't mean to harp on people who enjoy running or biking or hiking or walking; there is value in training for endurance as well. It's a matter of what kind of fitness goals you have, how much time you have, and how you want to look. Doing lower-impact exercise for longer periods of time will still help you lose some weight—it's just not the most efficient way to elevate your metabolism or build and maintain muscle. And when you don't en-gage all of your muscles, you end up with "lazy muscle"—underused muscle that has gone unchallenged (or underchallenged) for years and is therefore inefficient at doing pretty much everything, including burning fat.

Getting the body you've always wanted isn't about training longer. I'm going to show you the science-based shortcut to a better body, with workouts that take minutes, not hours. You'll pay your dues—it's not easy—but the return will leave you looking and feeling amazing, and that applies whether you're a fresh-out-of-college 20-something with all the time in the world to work out or a time-crunched 40-something juggling work, kids, and everything else life throws at you.

In just one 20-minute workout, you'll do your body more good than you could in some epic session on a stationary bike and the effects will stay with you for *days*, giving you more time to add back into work or play.

Here are some other perks of the 20-minute program:

• **MUSCLE MACHINERY UPGRADE:** Mitochondria are known as the powerhouses of our cells because they house most of your body's energy processes. And your muscles contain more mitochondria than any other part of your body! When you train hard, you increase the number of these cellular power factories in the muscle, so your body can use energy (i.e., stored fat) more efficiently. Generally, the greater the demand placed on working muscles, the more mitochondria are packed into your muscle. It's like replacing the fuel filter in your car: without even changing the octane you put in the tank, you get more mileage out of every gallon.

• **BETTER NUTRIENT DELIVERY:** All muscle is crisscrossed with blood vessels that help deliver oxygen and nutrients throughout the body. But did you know that you can increase the number of these tiny blood vessels that feed a muscle? According to a Danish study published in the *Journal of Physiology*,[2] high intensity interval training (HIIT) increased the number of blood vessels in muscle fibers after just a few weeks. This means that muscle is better conditioned, more resistant to fatigue, and generally better at shuttling fat and other fuel sources where they need to go to be burned: muscle cells!

• **A STRONGER LOOK:** You might think that you don't need to focus on strength to get leaner or healthier but you'd be wrong. Training against resistance—even if it's just gravity or your own bodyweight—not only builds bone density and streamlines muscle tissue but it's key for achieving that post-workout burn we've discussed. Muscles capable of handling more weight are usually better at helping you burn more fat. No need to bench-press a Smart Car. But if you're using superlight weights all the time and not compelling your muscles to work harder, then you're shortchanging how much fat you can burn overall. Don't let people tell you that training muscle will make you bulky or heavier—that's nonsense.

FAT FACT: Here's further motivation to start swapping fat for muscle: Claude Bouchard, an obesity researcher from the Pennington Biomedical Research Center, revealed that **a pound of muscle, at rest, burns about six calories per day**.[3] Compare that with a pound of fat, which burns about two. This means that **muscle is three times more metabolically active than fat.**

• **DIABETES-PROOFING:** Numerous studies have demonstrated that increasing the amount of lean muscle mass in your body helps to *improve* insulin sensitivity, or your body's ability to handle this crucial hormone. That is to say that it improves your body's ability to deal with carbs, reducing the crazy spikes in insulin from your pancreas which can result in fat storage. These "spikes" come from eating processed carbohydrates as well as foods rich in healthy carbs like whole-grain breads, lentils, fruits, and certain grains. So again, having active, hard-charging metabolic muscle can help you stay lean and, in this case, reduce your risk of diabetes.[4, 5]

METABOLIC MUSCLE PITFALLS

Now that you know what metabolic muscle is, it will be easier to grasp how to train it, eat for it, and think about how you want your body to change. Bodies have only so much real estate, making the way you choose to occupy that space all the more important. A body that has a higher proportion of hardworking (metabolic) muscle has the best chance of producing the long-lasting lean that you're looking for. When fat starts to creep up, your body becomes less efficient at, well, everything. Unhealthy levels of body fat are associated with higher levels of chronic disease than lower body fat percentages.

Compromising the body's ability to maintain muscle spells disaster for anyone seeking total-body change. So now that you know that the goal is to create and maintain active, metabolic muscle, it should be easy to identify some of the reasons you may not have achieved your weight loss goals in the past.

Ask yourself: have you fallen into one of these traps?

1. CALORIE CUTTERS. *Calories in, calories out.* While it's true that many of us are just eating too much and that a reduction in calories will probably result in some weight loss, going too low can wreak havoc on your body's metabolism, hormone production, health, and performance. Super low-calorie diets also backfire because the body's built-in survival instinct kicks in when calories are too low and trigger it to store fat, because it doesn't know where its next meal is coming from. Adequate consumption of the right kinds of foods helps you to power through, and recover from, the workouts required to maximize metabolic muscle. Besides that, *not all calories are created equal.* You want to eat for nutrition and performance—not numbers.

WOMEN AND WEIGHT LIFTING: A BULKY PROBLEM

While it's not a common sight at most gyms, I'm sure you've seen some very athletic women with big, bulky muscles. Naturally, this has led many women to be wary of training with weights. The assumption is that any use of resistance will cause a gain of pounds and inches or that it could compromise the look they're going for.

I won't lie to you: it *is* possible to get bulky if you train the wrong way. Typically, this means increasingly heavy weights done with particular sets-and-reps schemes designed to build that kind of muscle. So it can happen, but it's just *not* an easy thing for women to do, so don't let that scare you away from strength training.

A little extra muscle isn't something to try to avoid at all costs, because it *can* help you burn more calories at rest. You don't have to worry, though, because that's not how we train here. I'm going to teach you how to lift the right way to burn more fat. You're going to develop a strong, athletic body that opens doors for you. When I'm done with you, you'll be able to choose nearly any physical goal and go after it with greater success.

2. CARDIO CRAZIES. Cardio is good. But you have to do the right type, at the right intensity, and for the right amount of time *if you want to get lean*. Just getting on a treadmill or bike and sweating for an hour can definitely help you lose some weight and do some good for your heart, but this can also cause loss of muscle tissue. As the body burns through its preferred fuel sources (stored carbs, then available fat), it goes on the hunt for additional kindling, usually in the form of your muscles' amino acid supply. Interval training at higher intensities, on the other hand, spares (and even strengthens) muscle, while increasing how much fat you can burn well after your workout.

3. LIGHT-WEIGHTS. Many of my female clients worry about lifting heavier weight out of fear of gaining pounds. So they stick to lighter weight at higher rep ranges in an effort to burn more calories, thinking that this will be the key to fat loss. But you have to stimulate muscle effectively in order to make it stronger and more active metabolically. People fall into the trap of lifting a weight 10 times when they could have lifted it 15–20 times or simply loaded more weight on the bar to begin with. You don't have to be a bodybuilder, but you do have to accept that (relatively) heavier weights and/or more reps are the best way to train your muscles for greater strength and fat loss. You can also challenge your muscles without lifting weights. In Chapter 11, I'll show you variations on common bodyweight exercises that dial up the intensity and create all the stimulus you need to get the results you want.

4. SHOWTIME TRAINERS. We're all training to look better but you're not going to get there just training "showtime" muscle, doing all curls, crunches, and kickbacks. These are all basically vanity workouts, with an aesthetics-driven focus. But the body is built to move in seven basic ways—squat, lunge, push, pull, twist, bend, and gait—at multiple joints at a time. These are the primal patterns that make up every human movement. And these are the movement patterns you need to focus on to get the most bang for your buck. That's exactly what we'll do in the next 20 days.

5. CARB HATERS. Contrary to what most people think, carbs aren't the devil. In fact, they are your body's favorite source of energy. When you cut carbs drastically, you can lose weight quickly but this is almost always water weight. Your body can eventually settle into a pattern of gradual weight loss but you will also be constantly yearning for carbs, and this yearning tends to spell disaster (i.e., bingeing) for most people. On top of that, your workouts—where you're working on improving your body's ability to burn fat at rest—are compromised because of a lack of available fuel. If you want to keep training the way you always have trained, then low-carb might work for you. But if you're reading this, then you're probably ready to step things up and I'm going to show you how to choose the right carbs, portions, and timing to support your workouts.

6. CARB LOVERS. Leaning on the "carbs are fuel" philosophy a little *too* heavily, some people think that indulging in all the carbs they want won't have any adverse effects. They'll just train it away, right? Wrong. There are a few problems with "carb loading." First, unless you are training for a triathlon, you're never going to get through *all* of your carb stores. Second, higher consumption of carbs as a rule will most likely lead to the consumption of more *bad* carbs, the type that digest quickly in the body, causing rapid rises in insulin, which prompts the body to store fat. Not all carbs are created equal, so ditch the bad ones and focus on the good.

7. FAT PHOBICS. "*If I eat fat, I'll get fat.*" This oft-repeated refrain needs to be put to bed. Your body needs this crucial nutrient to support joint health and heart function, get glowing skin, and absorb many essential vitamins and minerals in your food. You just can't go overboard or eat the wrong fats. At nine calories per gram (compared to four calories for carbs and protein), fat is the most energy-dense of all the macronutrients. Many people think cutting out fat is an easy way to cut pounds. But this creates a whole different set of problems and still deprives your body of a crucial food source. Some fats—like those from nuts, seeds, coconuts, and avocados—are actually great for your health *and* your weight loss efforts. There will be much more on this later, as well.

8. OVERDOERS. If you're someone who likes to train hard by day and hit the town by night, you may be in for a rude awakening. Allowing your body to recover from your workouts with adequate sleep is vital. Remember, the workout is just the stimulus. Your body actually changes during rest and recovery. Without sufficient rest, your body increases production of a stress hormone called cortisol, which can actually eat away at muscle tissue and cause you to accumulate belly fat. Yikes.

The next 20 days are going to teach you to avoid these common missteps. Day by day, you'll develop better training, nutritional habits, and mental habits that will have you speeding toward your best body ever.

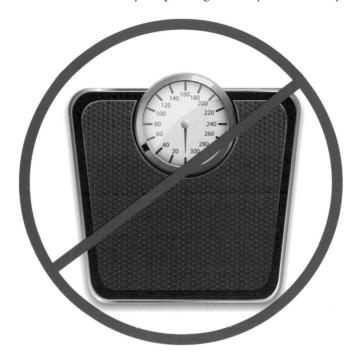

DITCH THE SCALE

Over the next 20 days we will build a formula and an appetite for success that will never leave you. But if you expect to keep on the path to long-lasting, total-body change, you need to choose the right measures of success.

Let's be clear: the scale is *not* the best indicator of your progress when you're trying to get fitter and leaner. In fact, I wouldn't put the scale second or even third on a list of performance indicators in a weight loss program. When you start a new exercise program, your muscles often accumulate fluid as a result of acute (temporary) inflammation. It's not uncommon for you to see a subtle increase in weight after one or two tough workouts! Your muscles are broken down by "microtrauma" (see page 67) through exercise, and even though continued exercise will result in lower overall levels of inflammation everywhere, this initial swelling—which may not be noticeable in the mirror—causes people to think that their workouts are failing them.

But that's just in the beginning. In the days and weeks that follow, the scale may produce other aberrations that are discouraging. Hard-training men, once they find their stride on a new program, may see a drop in weight that they categorize as too rapid, so they back off for fear of losing muscle, not realizing that their body has actually started digging into unseen fat stores.

After a few weeks on a workout plan, women may plateau for a short time before seeing the scale start to creep up again. This is usually attributable to a simple swap: muscle for fat.

In both cases, even though the mirror usually offers a good and honest reflection of their progress, they rely on the scale. Better indicators—and there are many—include how your clothes fit (which indicates loss of inches), the mirror, and other subtle cues such as better sleep, increased energy, improved mood, more mental sharpness, and just a better quality of life. **Repeat after me: Do not be a slave to the scale**. Think "waist loss," measured in inches—not weight loss, measured in pounds.

Right now, you're in the first stage of a beautiful metamorphosis. This 20-day transformation will be governed not by outside forces but by *you*. By making the commitment to developing metabolic muscle through a winning mindset, stepped-up workouts, and smarter eating, you're going to set yourself up for dramatic, long-term transformation. This is a much more effective strategy than simply trying to starve yourself down to a lower weight or sit on a stationary bike for an hour a day.

With the *20-Minute Body*, you'll have a leaner, stronger, and more sculpted physique. You're going to melt away inches (and pounds), drop sizes, and crush workouts that used to crush you. You're going to have a body full of muscle that works for you, and not just while you're grinding through a workout. Building metabolic muscle rewires your body to be more efficient at using (and producing) energy, while stoking the fire of your fat-fighting furnace.

Metabolic muscle is everything. It's not about working out for hours—you can get greater results in just minutes! Success is measured not in pounds but in inches. This paradigm shift is the beginning of a beautiful new you and I'm so excited to see your transformation. Let's get started.

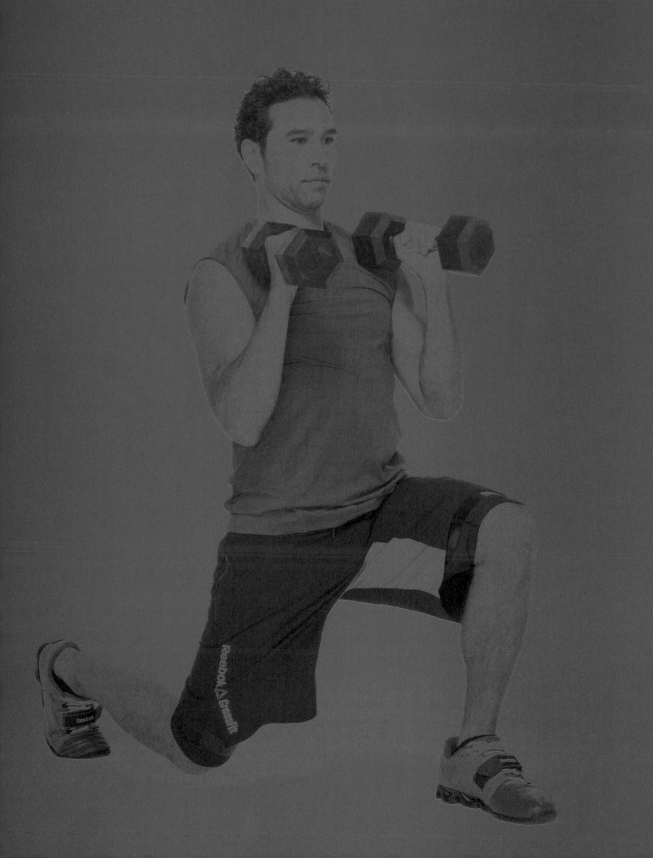

TWO

You Can Lose 20 Inches in Just 20 Minutes . . . Really

THE ECONOMY AND EFFICIENCY OF LOSING INCHES

KNOW WHAT YOU'RE THINKING: *What could I possibly get done in 20 minutes?* To most, the idea of a 20-minute workout delivering major results probably sounds like another in a long line of gimmicky fitness promises—the kind that have left you scratching your head and grabbing a pair of roomy sweatpants. Look, I get it. I've been a very vocal critic of these kinds of programs because they don't produce real results and sometimes they can do more harm than good. But I give you my word right up front: the programs in this book are based on years of experience, and hours of real-life testing on real-life people with real-life schedules.

I wouldn't ask you to do anything that I haven't done myself. No, let me go a step further: I wouldn't ask you to do anything that I wouldn't ask my friends and family to do. In fact, they were part of my test group!

When I first floated the 20-minute idea to friends and close clients, there were a few shrugs. *Okay, Brett.* But when I said that I could create a program that would allow people to lose 20 inches in 20 days with daily 20-minute commitments to training, food, and mental focus, I got laughs. Now it definitely sounded like a gimmick to them!

Part of me was offended but another part of me—the part that has helped change the lives of clients that other people thought were beyond help—wanted to prove them wrong. So I decided that I was going to just throw it down and have them try it. I knew that they would come away convinced. So why was I so confident?

Well, for one, I knew the short-burst workouts were built in a way that would force participants' bodies to respond very quickly. And one of the main obstacles for people, food planning, could be made easy if I provided them with healthy, flavorful, ingredient-minimal recipes. I also knew from personal experience that dedicating a few minutes a day to sharpening one's mental focus was the ingredient that many people were missing—the element that builds consistency in healthy living. Once people tie all of this together, it's not unreasonable to expect a loss of 20 inches *or more* in 20 days *or less.*

And how did my loved ones fare once they put the *20-Minute Body* principles to the test?

The proof is in the pictures (you can check them out at bretthoebel .com). They've lost *an average of* more than 20 inches and experienced significant weight loss as well, all in a single 20-day cycle, just by following the concepts laid out here. They're happier, healthier, and fitter than ever. Some of them achieved the weight loss they wanted in a single 20-day cycle. Others—especially those with a little more weight to lose—

did more than one 20-day cycle and, to this day, are seeing results well beyond the promise on the cover of this book.

So yeah, really. It's possible. Some A-listers and frequently photographed folks rely on the *20-Minute Body* program, but far and away, the biggest group that has seen results that transcend the scale consists of people just like you: busy moms and time-crunched executives, lifetime exercisers who've hit a plateau, and those returning from a long layoff. Everyone who has tried this recalibration becomes hyper-fit and hyper-motivated to stay that way. It's empowering when you realize how fast and how *much* this focused, time-saving approach can actually change how you look, feel, and think.

Wondering what a 20-minute time investment really looks like? Read on.

20-MINUTE WORKOUTS

This is the part of the *20-Minute Body* that raises the most eyebrows for some reason when, in reality, it is the most thoroughly researched. First of all, there's the mental part of it. We tend to get bored by our workouts if they are too long and just do them on automatic pilot. But studies have shown that most people are able to maintain strong concentration for up to 20 minutes. The mind, like muscle, fatigues and starts performing tasks less efficiently after 20 minutes.[6] So the 20-minute duration of these workouts (some will be slightly shorter) means that you are capable of pouring every bit of your mental stock into your physical performance.

But while 20 minutes is a sweet spot when it comes to training, I am not so rigid or so stubborn as to think it's the only one. Because when it comes to training, all the studies in the world won't matter if you can't get your clients to keep doing it. You might have a 5-minute workout that produces great results, but if your clients won't do it day in and day out, then what's the point? So I wanted actual, real-time feedback from people to see what time commitment worked best.

So, using workout guidelines that fit within certain time frames—10–15 minute workouts were jam-packed and intense, while 30 minute workouts had the intensity spread out a bit but involved more total work—I observed what I could and talked to everyone afterward.

Not surprisingly, I found that the people in the shorter workouts—even though they were huffing and puffing—didn't feel they were getting much done. Even though it was a hard-core metabolic blast, in most cases, they still had energy left in the tank. They told me that they could have kept going a bit longer.

The ones in the 30-minute groups started trailing off after 15–20 minutes. Their form started getting sloppy and they seemed to lose interest. Afterward, they said that the workout went on too long and that while they felt strong at the beginning, they couldn't do it every day. My older sister, in particular, shared with me that 30-minute workouts, because of prep time, made her have to get up an hour earlier (for morning workouts) or stay up an hour later (for nighttime workouts). Neither one of those formats was going to work. A slightly shorter workout would give her more leeway and make it easier to manage her time.

Lightbulb. It was time to try the 20-minute window.

Again, the workouts were high on relative intensity, so you'd expect people to fall off. But they didn't. In fact, despite the uptick in difficulty, people stayed engaged for the full 20 minutes. Turns out, the people who didn't feel that 10–15 minutes were long *enough* were plenty satisfied by just adding a few more productive minutes. The people that we normally lost halfway through the 30-minute workouts kept it up because they felt 20 minutes were just easier to keep up—they could see the light at the end of the tunnel, so they were comfortable pushing harder.

As a result, both groups got better results! It was like the story of the Three Bears: one workout length was too hot, one was too cold, but the 20-minute length was just right.

To get the most out of a 20-minute session, you have to commit to stepping things up a bit. You don't have to be a hurricane of body parts on Day 1, but you definitely need to be willing to work at a higher level than you normally do. Research shows that training with high-intensity intervals—several tough bouts of work, each followed by a short recovery period—increases fat-burning at rest while preserving and strengthening muscle and in far less time. And as we've discussed, this type of training also helps you to burn more calories after your workout. Considering all that, it's easy to understand why this recipe for getting lean has almost universally replaced most traditional gym routines.

But the upside doesn't stop there. The benefits of 20-minute workouts are amazing, not just because they favor high-intensity work, but because people will *continue to do them!*

You might not feel you can do the intense 60- or 90-minute workouts that you see advertised on TV, but 20? Come on, your favorite sitcom has an actual run time of 22 minutes (I'm going to assume you fast-forward through commercials the way I do)! You can move your body for that long if it means a mind-blowing, total-body makeover in 20 days.

20-MINUTE MEALS

Without question, the toughest part of any weight loss program is the nutrition. There are so many things working against you when it comes to eating right, but one of the greatest factors is time. It takes time to shop, it takes time to set out the food you're going to prepare, it takes time to cut veggies and prep meat, and it takes time to cook and clean it all up. These are all very real challenges, no doubt about it. So I thought it was time that we adapted. It may have been the trickiest part of the *20-Minute Body* but, with the help of my good friend, celebrity chef Rocco Whalen, we've removed all of the roadblocks. Your food, like your fitness, can be addressed in 20 minutes *flat.*

Some drive-thrus take longer than that! But you can create tasty, wholesome, and healthy meals in less than 20 minutes. Our idea of how good food is prepared is sometimes skewed, isn't it? There's the leisurely pace of shows on the Food Network where the hosts don't seem to have a care in the world, tossing in perfectly portioned bowls of this and that, sipping wine, and chatting to the camera. Then there are the hard-core shows that give you a peek behind the curtain of busy restaurant kitchens, where fire and passion and chaos churn out award-worthy dishes for innocent, oblivious patrons. Does either of these kitchens look like yours?

No. In most kitchens, the only chaos is created by hungry families and approaching bedtimes and the wine is used to drown it all out! We have so many other commitments over the course of a day, the last thing we want to think about is the chore of prepping meals—let alone "healthy" ones.

I'm as much a novice in the kitchen as anyone. I don't have Rocco's knife skills and I couldn't tell you much about red wine reductions or homemade glazes. In fact, the more ingredients there are, the more discouraged I become. That's why these recipes are really simple. They're ingredient-minimal. In many cases, the work of chopping vegetables and preparing proteins takes 5 minutes or less. The slow-cooker recipes almost cook themselves, they're so easy. And in this book I've given you lots of ideas for how to use one key ingredient to make several different meals so that you can "batch cook" your protein and spend even less time in the kitchen.

Chef Rocco lost more than 100 pounds while continuing his day job as a professional chef running several booming restaurants. He understands firsthand how to make meals that are both healthy and delicious, as well as how to fit his workouts into his hectic schedule. His recipes take just 20 minutes or less to prepare, so you won't be slaving away in the kitchen for hours on end. Together we've created dozens of original recipes to fit your lifestyle. They'll help you to learn the *fastest* way to clean up your nutrition while enjoying your food. Weight loss happens fastest when you get your nutrition right, so Chef Rocco and I have developed menu plans that take all the guesswork out of fueling your body.

It really is a life-changing revelation when you realize that eating healthy food every day doesn't take an unlimited amount of time and money! Once you start cranking these meals out in minutes, you'll realize that you're closer to your ideal body than you've ever been.

20-MINUTE MINDSET

Many things can derail your success when it comes to getting fit. But it's my firm belief that your mind can be your greatest enemy in your quest to become healthier, which is why your success over the next 20 days—or even the next 20 years—is wholly dependent on making it your greatest ally. The good news is that you can whip your gray matter into shape, so to speak, in as little as 20 minutes a week (more if you have time to spare). Remember *fitness from within*? This is where it's forged.

If you're reading this right now, then chances are you've fought tooth and nail to arrange this little retreat—this moment away from your phone, your kids, your computer screen, and your job. That's because life is awash with distractions that can prevent you from reaching your goals. While so many start out strong in new fitness programs, they quickly find that the mind fatigues well before the body.

That's why the mindset training is so important and not just for the short term. It's important to incorporate these new habits for life, so you should be mentally prepared to persevere through discouragement, fatigue, and other challenges. How is this achieved? Through a little old-fashioned "Me Time"—a daily, minutes-long block of time committed to focusing on you. It's a time to drown out the distractions of the day, to notice the changes you're experiencing, to make note of your successes, and to set yourself up for another great day tomorrow.

In the grand scheme of this program, this window of time is the third, final, and most decisive commitment you can make. And you should keep this commitment to yourself whether you have a single, solid block of time (I know this can be hard to find), or whether you have to break it up into multiple sessions. Since we're fans of intervals, you can divide your mindset training into a few minutes in the morning and a few in the evening if that works better for you. By week's end, if you're in the ballpark of 20 minutes, you will have done more to cement your goals than most other weight loss hopefuls.

The mindset training allows you to focus on your "why"—your ultimate motivation for getting healthy, lean, and strong. This can be done through exercises like journaling or active breathing or more passive practices like simple quiet reflection, so long as you're keeping your focus on strengthening your commitment to yourself.

If you've tried to lose weight before, then you know that a rough day, a bad phone call, fatigue, and feelings are all diet killers. Having the right frame of mind and committing to fitness within is too important *not* to work on. And this, like the fitness and nutrition parts of this program, is not a burdensome pursuit. Just minutes a day—striving for 20 per week—is all it takes to build the inner muscle that will carry you for the next 20 days and beyond.

THE 20-MINUTE PROMISE

If you are making these 20-minute commitments—daily 20-minute workouts, 20-minute meals, and 20 minutes per week of mindset training —you'll be speeding toward your goals, and the mirror and tape measure will tell the tale. The hustle and bustle of everyday living may have you convinced that you don't have time to get healthy, but I'm here to tell you that you do. Twenty minutes is the secret sauce for fitness, food, and focus. In all three areas, 20 minutes works for many reasons.

So anyone who tells you that you need to work out longer or take more steps in the kitchen, or that mental focus requires more time, is either not in touch with the realities of real-life schedules, or trying to get more money out of you, or both.

When you drop 20 inches in 20 days, you'll understand just what power there is in these 20-minute daily time commitments.

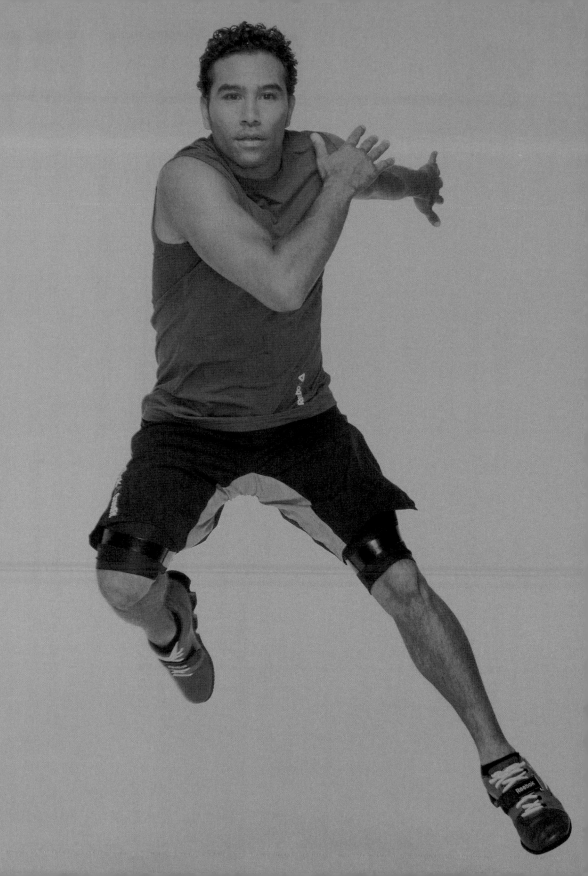

THREE

Busting the Cardio Myth

EVERY DAY, MILLIONS OF AMERICANS stroll into gyms and take their places on "cardio row," the long line of treadmills, stair-climbers, exercise bikes, and ellipticals that are part of any gym-scape. The draw to these machines is epidemic. The best evidence of this is the fact that there are special rules to govern their use, such as:

Do not use for more than 30 minutes if someone is waiting.

Oh, the humanity. And if you've ever seen the indignant looks of those waiting in the wings, or heard the ranting of people who have had to "cut their workout short," then you know this is a very real problem. During rush hour in a gym—usually 7–9 in the morning and again between 5 and 7 at night—these machines are first come, first served and countless gym beefs have started within these disputed territories. People rearrange work schedules and take dicey shortcuts on their commutes to the gym in order to stake their claim to their favorite machine before anyone else.

And astonishingly, those who show up late seem to have no problem waiting, sometimes *over an hour*, to get onto a machine.

I don't fault either group (or the equipment). For as long as any of us can remember, cardio row has been regarded as the place you need to be if you want to shed a few pounds or look a little tighter. There's a great sense of reward when we see that calorie counter tick away, assigning a number to how "productive" a workout has been.

In my experience, the people who are fighting for time on these machines also fall into a few other camps. They rarely lift weights and when they do, it is usually very nonstructured. They believe in a "calories in, calories out" approach to fitness. They believe that if 20 minutes are good, then 40 minutes are better. And even the most dedicated cardio fanatics usually do the same program, on the same machine, at the same pace, for the same amount of time, day in and day out.

Those who train away from the gym can be guilty of the same things, taking a jog along the same trail at the same speed that they've been at for years, for example.

Those who live on cardio row make up a huge percentage of the exercising population of this country and maybe you're one of 'em. But if you look around, a singular truth stands out: if this approach were really working, we'd all be a lot thinner. Instead, obesity in this country is at an all-time high.

There's another fallout from the cardio-till-the-cows-come-home approach and it has to do with muscle. Hitting a 1-hour cardio class and doing a bit of weight training is admirable—certainly preferable to doing nothing at all—but it can lead to a very specific type of physique. Those who champion long, steady cardio sessions may end up losing some weight but are left looking less athletic than when they started, with less-than-impressive muscle and some lingering body fat. This look is referred to as "skinny fat" and it is all too common with many of the cardio crowd. In fact, if you cardio-train too long at a low intensity, your body can end up cannibalizing your hard-earned muscle for fuel!

So is cardio row completely useless? Should you be avoiding it? Or should we simply rethink how these pieces of equipment are used and apply a revamped approach to cardio for better results? These are the questions you should be asking. And once you have the answers, you'll never worry about that 30-minute time limit again. Why would you want to?

LONG AND SLOW VS. SHORT AND INTENSE

One of the biggest problems with cardio row is that it has come to be viewed as leisure . . . not work. I'm always amazed when I see people taking up these machines while talking on the phone, playing games on their tablets, or reading a magazine! This completely ignores the basic fact that you have to work hard to see results in anything you do but *especially* when it comes to fitness. Except for a very few genetically blessed individuals in this world, it takes serious effort to change your body. But the good news is that your body *wants* to be leaner, faster, and stronger and with the right program, it will respond like crazy. I hate to break it to you, but your 30-, 40- or 60-minute jaunts on the treadmill where you're pacing along at three miles per hour and fiddling with your iPhone will produce lackluster results.

If you're like my clients, you don't have a ton of time to devote to workouts like that. In fact, that may be why you've gained weight—you just don't think you have the time to work out. The good news about the workouts in this book is that they are very *dense*. You are literally getting more done for your body in about half the time of a normal workout. You get your engine all revved up for the day and it stays at that red line for a while, helping you to burn more calories while you're getting on with the business of life.

There are people who love to work out. I know because I'm one of them! Some people really enjoy zoning out on the elliptical for an hour. But the truth is, most of those folks can be doing better things with their time than continuing on with a workout that is less than effective for much longer than they need to. Workout efficiency is everything. When you're packing more work into less time, you're just getting more bang for your buck.

When you're willing to work hard, you can trigger real, lasting change within your body by actually spending *less* time training. Very few trainers are going to tell you to work out less. But that's exactly what I'm telling you to do.

Makes you rethink your approach a bit, huh?

Some people like to say to train harder, not smarter. Over the course of our 20-day window together, I'll help you understand why training harder *is* training smarter.

MAKING THE SHIFT

The "trade-off," if you will, with keeping your workouts to 20 minutes is that you have to be ready to dial things up a notch. You can definitely get more body benefits—longer calorie burn, better metabolism, better muscle tone—by training harder but the real strength for that kind of training comes from within.

Everything on this program will seem like a challenge at first. The mental training will feel awkward, the food corrections will be a bummer, and the workouts will be painful. But developing the intestinal fortitude to dig deep and take your body places it hasn't been in years (or ever), is a hurdle that you have to be willing to leap.

There will be times during these workouts when you start to doubt whether you can continue. But almost without fail, when I'm working with clients, I find that the mind gives out long before the body. And the only way to level that playing field is to build on successes. When you are huffing and puffing in the middle of one of my workouts in the first week, when you're ready to just shut it down because "Hey, nobody's watching anyway," remember the tough moments that you've already overcome to get here. Remember how your lungs were screaming at you on Day 4, but you pushed through and got up and got after it again the next day.

There will be plenty of fleeting moments, times when your brain just says "No, thanks," when it just doesn't want to give you what you need to push through. As you're working your body, remember that brain training is just as important. Focus your brain's attention on how you're going to look and feel afterward.

There are so many people who have below-average bodies because they put in a below-average effort day after day. Doing the same cardio session day in and day out is like lifting the same weight: you'll never get stronger. If you're training slowly, expect results to follow that pace. Just commit to working hard during your 20-minute workouts; enjoy moving your body a little harder than usual. If something feels too easy, then it probably is. Push a little harder until you feel a challenge. Over time, the harder workouts will get easier as you get stronger.

Pain is temporary. Health is forever. Push past your limits . . . once you go there, you'll never go back.

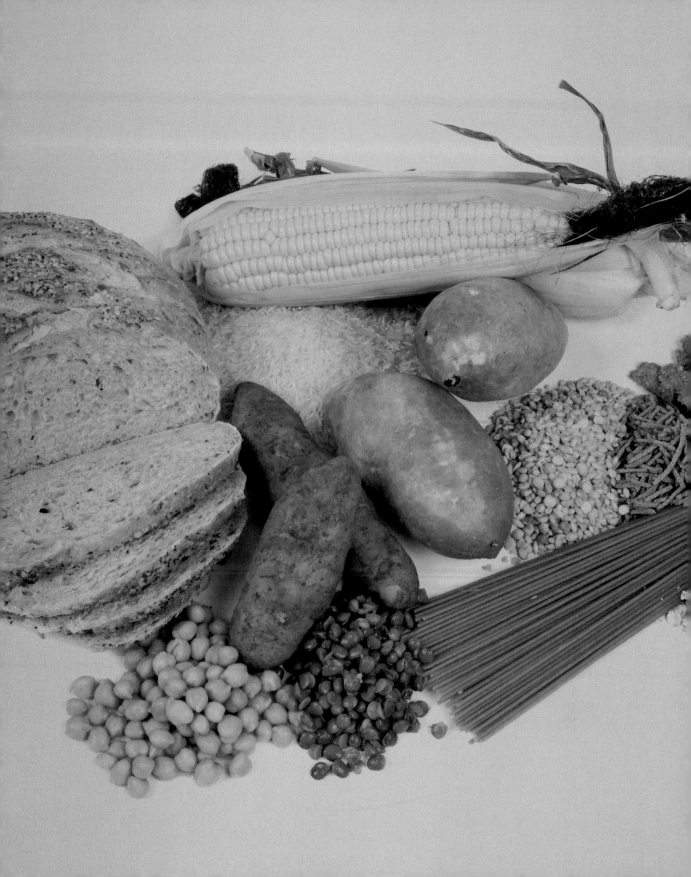

FOUR

Carb Amnesia

CHANCES ARE this isn't the first health or fitness book you've ever looked at. And I'm sure that you have friends who have tried to tell you what to do to lose weight, the latest diet or fitness plan that's worked for them. The info is everywhere, and it's often conflicting.

One of the areas of nutrition in which you'll find the most contradictory advice is carbohydrates. Many "experts" offer their views on carbs, but the most reputable and trustworthy sources have always said that carbs are fuel. That your body needs them. That your body *runs* on them.

But for most people, the concept of carbohydrates freaks them out so much that they often make bad decisions about what to eat when they're trying to lose weight. The kinds of decisions that actually lead to weight gain. They eat the wrong kinds of carbs and can't lose fat. Or they eat very few carbs but never seem to have any energy. Or they eat tons of good carbs, but can't seem to gain any muscle mass. All of these approaches can be catastrophic to your weight-loss efforts, leaving you backsliding and in worse shape than when you started.

Proper nutrition is *at least* 50 percent of the battle if you want to create fat-burning metabolic muscle, and an informed, healthy approach to carbs is a big part of that equation. You have to eat right. But you also have to eat delicious food, or else what's the point of eating healthfully at all?

Let's start off by seeing if you have Carb Amnesia, or another of the three carb traps I've identified below, and figure out how you can correct your thinking (and eating) when it comes to this powerful and essential macronutrient.

THE THREE CARB TRAPS

1. THE CARB-AMNESIAC: IT'S A CRUEL PHENOMENON. Carbs are energy, so when you're feeling sluggish, your brain convinces you that it's time to reach for some carbs. So you find yourself craving them constantly. You're doing one of two things to sabotage your diet. Either you're not planning your meals during the day and you're grabbing food wherever you can—food that very likely is loaded with the wrong types of carbs—or you *think* you're eating correctly, when in reality you're choosing carbs that move through your bloodstream very quickly, giving you a fast energy hit and then a major energy crash that leads you to eat more unhealthy carbs! Carb Amnesiacs have no idea how many carbs they're eating, or what those carbs are doing to their bodies. For example, many dieters grab rice cakes when they're hungry, not realizing that rice converts to sugar in the body faster than almost any other carb out there!

2. THE CARB JUNKIE: YOU'RE ALWAYS HUNGRY AND YOU DON'T KNOW WHY. But if I look in your lunch bag, I'm going to find things like crackers, pita chips, granola bars, energy bars, and sugar-dense foods like dried fruit. You don't eat enough protein—the fuel to create metabolic muscle. And you skimp on healthy fats because you think that "fat makes you fat." Nothing could be further from the truth—you'll learn more about that in Chapter 7. Bottom line: You're eating carbs only, and the wrong ones at that. You're a Carb Junkie!

3. THE CARB-O-PHOBE: YOU PROBABLY TRIED THE ATKINS DIET OR SOME VERSION OF IT A FEW YEARS AGO WHEN THE "EAT ALL THE PROTEIN AND FAT YOU WANT" FAD WAS MAKING THE ROUNDS. You won't eat even the healthiest carbs like fruit, fresh vegetables, and whole, fiber-packed grains, for fear they could ruin your get-lean efforts. You think the word "carb" can be universally replaced with "it's going to make me fat." Yet for all your forward thinking on the well-publicized dangers of carbs, you are still constantly lethargic, have a tough time maintaining mental focus and attention, don't have the gas to get through tough workouts, and tend to catch every cold that's going around. You're a Carb-o-Phobe!

Who's to blame for all the confusion about carbs? Honestly, it's us. The fitness industry throws the word "carb" around as though it's something to avoid at all costs. Or we talk about "carbs" as though that word applies *only* to processed grains and refined, added sugars—the kinds of carbs I definitely want you to avoid!

But the word "carb" by itself doesn't mean a food is healthy or un-healthy. Read on to discover what carbs actually are, why they're essential for your health, and how to eat the *right ones*. It's time to leave the carb traps behind and learn to make carbs work for you, not against you.

WHAT YOU *NEED* TO KNOW ABOUT CARBS

Carbs are one of the three macronutrients your body must be fed to function properly. The other two macronutrients are protein and fat. Carbs are the body's favorite source of energy for nearly every activity, including brain function, which is why people on low-carb diets tend to have a mental fog they can't seem to shake. Carbs are stored in your liver and in muscle tissue, and your body is always pulling from those caches to power activity. But when it comes to carbs, the type, the timing, and the amount go a long way toward determining what your body is going to do with that energy. So stay with me while we translate some science into service.

CARB TYPES MATTER

There are two very different kinds of carbohydrates running around out there, and you need to understand the difference between them in order to fuel your body properly.

SLOW-BURN BUFFET

Be fast to fill your plate with these slow-burning fuel choices:

Oatmeal

Sweet potatoes

Brown rice

Quinoa

High-fiber veggies (broccoli, leafy
    greens, carrots, beets)

Lentils

Chickpeas

Black beans

1. *Complex*—or *slow-fueling, slow-burning*—carbohydrates are carbs that take real time and energy to digest in your body. Slow-fueling carbs are made primarily of fiber or starch. They're normally found in a natural, unprocessed state.

Slow-fueling carbs don't just hit your bloodstream at full throttle. Instead, your body needs to burn energy to digest them, a process called *thermogenesis*. Slow-fueling carbs can be found in foods like fruit, vegetables, unprocessed grains (like quinoa), and some starches (like sweet potatoes). These kinds of foods are hard to overeat for a reason: they contain fiber. Try overdoing it on oatmeal sometime and you'll know what I'm talking about. Because of their slow-digesting, slow-absorbing properties, which leave you feeling fuller longer, these carbs are usually referred to as "good" carbs.

2. *Simple*—or *fast-fueling, fast-burning*—carbohydrates are carbs that enter your bloodstream quickly, giving you a quick "energy hit." Simple carbs include refined flours and added sugars. Most people who overdo it on simple carbs load up on things like white bread, white pasta, soda, and candy. Added simple carbs hide in many other foods, too (like the sugars in "healthy" granola bars and even pasta sauce).

Fast-fueling carbs are the kinds of carbs that can be way too easy to overindulge in, and most processed foods have tons of them. Processed carbs—the ones that are most likely to have added sugars, empty calories that don't fill you up, and other unhealthy additives like too much salt—are way too cheap and easy to find in our culture. You really have to work hard to avoid them. And because they have drastic impact on blood sugar and the hormones that regulate hunger, you have to be much more careful when consuming them. Hence, they are typically referred to as "bad" carbs.

FIBER IS YOUR FRIEND

Fiber helps to slow digestion and absorption of foods, so that they have a lesser impact on blood sugar. It also makes you feel fuller longer. A 2009 study[7] in the journal *Appetite* compared the satiety or fullness factor of apples, applesauce, and apple juice with added fiber before lunch. People who ate an apple before lunch ate 15 percent fewer calories than those who ate the applesauce or drank apple juice. This suggests that the fiber in the whole apple was more filling even when compared with the juice that had added fiber. Here are some ways to make sure you're getting enough:

- Eat whole fruits instead of drinking fruit juice.

- Snack on raw veggies, which have more fiber than cooked veggies.

- Make vegetables (your greens) half of your plate at every meal.

- Start the day with steel-cut oatmeal topped with higher-fiber fruit.

- Eat more beans.

- Eat only unprocessed grains, and limit your serving sizes.

On the basis of this knowledge, you've probably figured out that slow-fueling carbs will be the most-used source of energy on the *20-Minute Body* program. But I say *most*-used source . . . not the only used source. And there's a reason for that.

CARB TIMING MATTERS

Slow-fueling carbs give you a steady stream of energy and help to keep your blood sugar in check. There is no quick energy hit, no energy "high" to come down off. These types of carbs are what you want in the tank to sustain you through your daily activity, and having enough of them ensures that your stored fuel (glycogen) is topped off as you head into workouts. Because they are released slowly, slow carbs are the ideal choice for breakfast, when you want to fuel up for the day ahead. But that same slow trickle, which barely makes a dent in blood sugar, also makes slow-fueling carbs a good choice at other times of the day, such as between meals or in the afternoon to forestall that post-lunch crash By slowing digestion, you reduce the impact of carbs on your body.

So, clearly, they have an edge over fast-fueling carbs, right? Most of the time, yes. But fast-fueling carbs—when you choose the right ones—have some very specific benefits that you should also be aware of.

When your body is screaming for quick nutrition, these carbs are digested and absorbed quickly, flooding your bloodstream with energy and forcing your body to make a decision on what to do with it. If you're about to work out, great—it will send that fuel directly to muscles for use. But if you're sitting on your can in your cubicle, then your body doesn't have that advantage. Instead, it decides to store the energy away for later use, but not before leaving you with an unwanted spike in blood sugar and a post-carb fatigue that'll have you searching for a pillow.

So the best times to eat simple carbs would be an hour or so before a workout and in the minutes immediately following a workout. In the first instance, your body can quickly digest, absorb, and utilize the fuel in these carbs, which can translate directly into energy for training. Immediately post-workout, your body is low on stored sugar, and those fast-fueling carbs go immediately to replenish this supply while also spiking key hormones in your body that maximize recovery.

But you still have to choose the right ones—no candy bars masquerading as "sports nutrition bars" for you. The processed carbs from such sources are more likely to end up on your butt or waistline than back in your liver or muscle cells and are usually combined with other unhealthy additives like heaps of salt and fillers. Better choices include fruits or fruit juices that are higher in that fast fuel like figs, cantaloupe, or pineapple.

But remember, the timing is everything. If you have these foods too far ahead of a workout, the energy from the sugar will go unused and will be stored by your body. Wait too long after your workout and the sugar doesn't have the same effect on recovery. You end up with the blood sugar spike without any of the advantage. So for the fast-fueling carbs, keep it to 30–60 minutes before or after workouts.

> SMART CARB TIP: You'll notice on this diet that you are always pairing a protein with your carbs. That's because protein causes an even slower uptake of those carbs, meaning less of an impact on your blood sugar. Protein takes longer to digest than carbs, so the inclusion of protein in most meals and snacks help to ensure slower, steadier digestion. And that's a good thing, because when you digest slowly, you won't experience those insulin surges that prompt your body to store fat!

CARB AMOUNTS MATTER

So we know that carb types matter. Fast-burning carbs affect the body differently from slow-burning carbs. We also know that carb timing matters. You want slow-burning carbs early to power your day and fast-burning carbs to provide a quick energy hit before workouts and to fuel your recovery when they are over. But your control of carbohydrates doesn't end there. Even though "good" carbs exist, you can still get too much of a good thing.

Too much of any kind of fuel in your body gets turned into fat. Slow-burning carbs like quinoa and black beans, if eaten to excess, will leave your body with more fuel than it can handle at one time. Even if you're diligently performing your workouts, overconsumption of slow-burning carbs will end up causing your body to store some of it. So just choosing sweet potatoes over regular potatoes doesn't give you license to have four of them at dinner. You can't eat a loaf of whole wheat bread and expect it to be fine because whole wheat is "slow-burning." Same goes for all of those healthy baked goods made without white flour—they are not an invitation to eat five cookies without consequences. Excess food invariably leads to excess weight.

The same principle applies with fast-burning carbs, which can be even more disastrous. Not only will excess simple carbs be stored as fat, but the immediate impact on your body is drastic. Fast-burning carbs spike your blood sugar, causing your body to release more of the hormone insulin. Insulin, sadly, signals your body to store fat. It's a nasty cycle and fast-burning carbs are a nasty instigator. After it spikes, your blood sugar drops through the basement, and your hormones signal your brain to get more food . . . so you go rummaging for more. Also, these carbs don't leave you with the same sense of fullness, so they lead you to eat more. This is why many people feel full on a modest slice of watermelon but can take down a half dozen cupcakes in one sitting.

THE 411 ON FRUIT

Technically, fruit contains fast-burning carbs because it contains two types of sugars: glucose and fructose. Glucose is stored in your muscles as glycogen, an easily accessed source of energy that is released for fuel when needed. Fructose cannot be readily used by your body and has to first travel to your liver to be converted into glucose. But fruit in its natural state (not dried and sweetened, and definitely not stuffed into a Thanksgiving pie!) is also full of fiber, so it takes time to digest and makes you feel satisfied for a long time. Plus it has tons of vitamins and antioxidants in it—all of the good stuff. Bottom line: Don't avoid fruit because you think it has too much sugar in it, but don't eat fruit at every meal, either.

HOW TO MANAGE CARBS

Truth: Carbs are muscle fuel. Without carbs, you won't have the energy to get through the workouts I've designed for you. If you're avoiding them, you're probably tired all the time because you're not giving your brain and body the fuel they need to function. And if you're eating too many carbs (or too many of the wrong type), you're probably not getting enough of the other nutrients you need for your body to function well, either.

Here's a test. After a big carb meal, check in with yourself an hour later. How do you feel? Did you react positively or negatively to what you ate? If you're having a positive reaction, you'll feel satisfied, energetic, and good. Bad reactions are real simple: you're still hungry, still having cravings, bloated, belching; you have a stomachache; you're drowsy; and you can't focus. If you feel any of those symptoms, then it's time to go back and look at your carbohydrate type, timing, and amount from that meal. As I said, carbs can work for you or against you.

With this guide, however, you can finally start to get a handle on carbs. They're a food source to be managed, not omitted. They're to be enjoyed but within reason. When you notice how you feel by using a more balanced approach to all food, carbs included, you'll stick with the changes you've made.

THE ECONOMY OF HEALTH

We're all used to eating a certain way and, unfortunately, processed carbs are everywhere. They're in everything. Processed carbs are cheap. But healthy carbs are affordable, too. You can get a bag of brown rice for $2. A few pounds of oatmeal can be had for under $4. A $10 investment in fresh veggies will last a family of four well over a week. Swapping out your bad carbs for good ones isn't as difficult as you might think, it's just different. And it will cost you much less in the long run than eating takeout or fast food, while also reducing your overall health expenses. Basically, it costs you more *not* to eat this way!

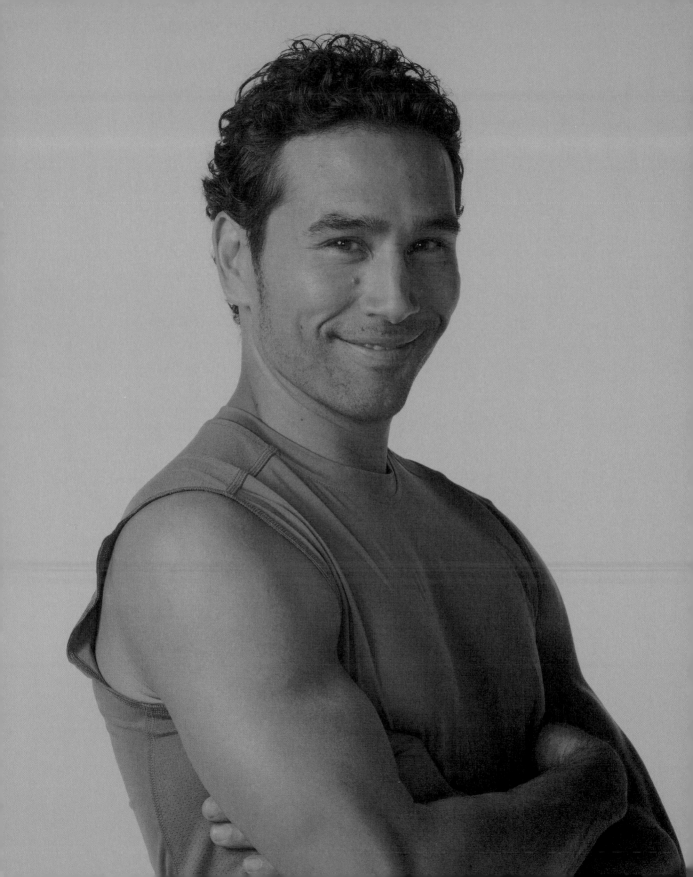

FIVE

The 20-Minute Mindset

W HEN WE START working out together in Chapter 11, we will pay close attention to repetitions: the more reps you do, the more skilled and efficient your body becomes at executing a given movement. And the more efficient you are at that movement, the stronger you become. But this type of adaptation isn't exclusive to your muscle. It can be just as readily applied to your mind.

In high school, when I had finally committed to getting healthier, it took just as many mental reps as physical ones to get to where I wanted to be. Every time a coach told me to do 10 push-ups, I'd tell myself I needed to do 20. And I would. Every time I found myself rummaging through the pantry to satisfy a craving, I'd tell myself to seek out a healthier snack. And I would. These mental reps were incredibly important because each time I pushed through a bit of discomfort or resisted a sugary craving, it became easier to do it the next time, and the next. That's because the behaviors we repeat most often become imprinted onto our neural pathways. The repetition builds strength of resolve, in much the same way that physical repetitions strengthen neural connections. Interestingly, beginners in the weight room gain strength rapidly, not because of an increase in muscle size but because the brain is actively learning the new movement patterns that new trainees are performing. The brain's learning computer is the most powerful asset for physical improvement.

Mental reps are an essential part of this program because they make your mind stronger. That's why you're going to devote several minutes a day to developing the proper mindset, with the goal of devoting 20 minutes per week. That's not much to ask, is it? It averages out to less than three minutes a day. Twenty minutes over the course of the week, stealing moments here and there, will help to make sure your weight loss plan becomes a mental habit, not a daily struggle. Of the three components of this program, your mental training is the least time intensive but perhaps the most important. It is crucial for your overall success.

Why commit only 20 minutes a week to mental training if it's so important? Well, for one thing, I want to give you a time goal that is manageable. Just as with your workouts or your food prep, if I asked you to do it for 40 or even 60 minutes a day, I'd probably lose you. You are welcome to commit more than 20 minutes weekly, if you can.

I guarantee that if you hit (or exceed) that 20, you're going to be so much stronger in your food and your fitness. A tiny investment in yourself each day can have a tremendous impact on your life.

THE ELEMENTS OF MINDSET TRAINING

When you train your body, different exercises focus on different muscle groups. Squats hit your legs pretty hard, while push-ups zero in on your chest and shoulders. Training each area individually is good, but if you want total-body results, then you have to train your total body. When you're doing your mindset training, there are also different areas that require individual attention. By working on these separate areas, you build a mind that is strong enough to fend off any temptation, and persevere through any workout—a mind that is able to develop healthy habits and maintain the commitment you've made to your body.

So let's look at a few mental exercises that target specific mental resources: choosing mantras, dealing with chatter, and finding your "why."

MANTRAS

I'm a huge believer in the power of mantras to inspire results, whether it's in the gym, at work, or in your personal life. A mantra is simply a word or phrase that is repeated often, and it is usually an expression of an intention or a belief. Find a mantra each week that expresses the deepest idea about what you want to achieve, and repeat it—silently or audibly—as often as you can in order to reinforce that concept. It can be funny, serious, inspirational, or reflective. It's meant to be an expression of your own personality. Make sure it's fresh, has real energy, and inspires you to give your all each day for the next 20 days . . . and beyond.

When you choose your mantra, write it down and post it where you're going to see it a lot. It could be a screen saver on your computer or phone, taped to a corkboard in your office, or posted on your bathroom mirror so that you see it first thing in the morning.

These don't have to be Shakespearean, just simple and meaningful to you. One of my favorite mantras is actually: "Movement, music, and mantra." Those are the three things that get me going in the morning and remind me of what I have to do to have a productive day. I have to commit to moving my body, I need my tunes to keep me motivated, and I have to dial in to my personal mantra to make sure I'm going in the right direction. All three of these ideas are key for getting and keeping a positive mindset.

I've listed 20 mantras on the following page that my clients have come up with to keep themselves going. You'll see that some of them are geared to help them deal with the challenges of specific workouts, some deal with accountability, and some are reminders to stay tough. These things are personal to each client. They are mantras that are specific to each person's mental hurdles. Feel free to use one of these yourself until you can think of one that is more specific to your goals:

1. I am the sum total of my thoughts.

2. Squats make the world a better place.

3. Just keep going, no matter what.

4. It's the "start" that stops most people.

5. Pain is temporary, health is forever.

6. Don't wait until you've reached your goal to be proud of yourself.

7. I am stronger than my excuses.

8. You never know how strong you are, until being strong is the only choice you have.

9. Progress, not perfection.

10. I'd rather be sore today than sorry tomorrow.

11. Exercise changes everything.

12. Good things come to those who work their butts off.

13. If you want it, work for it.

14. Suck it up now and you won't have to suck it in later.

15. I don't stop when I'm tired; I stop only when I'm done.

16. The separation is in the preparation.

17. Sweat with soul!

18. Life begins outside your comfort zone.

19. My biggest risk may be the one I didn't take.

20. I trust myself to fight for what I want.

You might think some of these mantras are silly at first glance. You might think that their value is tough to quantify or that they don't really have a measurable effect on changing your body. You'd be wrong. I've seen over the years just how powerful these mantras can be and how they add up to more reps completed, more inches lost, and more pounds shed. Your mantras may very well be a key factor determining how well you do in the next 20 days and well after that.

NIXING NEGATIVE CHATTER

We've all heard it before—that little voice in your head that tells you that your body needs a break before a set is done, that whispers that the dessert or the extra drink isn't going to kill you. Chatter is like static that interrupts your picture of a healthier lifestyle, because it prompts you to slow down, to quit, or to settle. And it always shows up when you need it the least, doesn't it? It is always loudest when you're on that last round of a workout, when your alarm goes off at 6 a.m., or when you encounter some leftover dessert from your kid's class party.

> *Don't overdo it and hurt yourself.*
> *You could use some more sleep anyway.*
> *One bite. Just one.*

It's like the little animated cartoon devil on your shoulder telling you what you *can't* do, or feeding you reasons why you *don't* need to do something that you had carefully and intentionally planned to do. Chatter is especially insistent when it comes to tackling things that you know will be difficult . . . things like working through a new, 20-day fitness plan! It preys upon the very weaknesses you are trying to snuff out.

The best way to keep chatter in check is to have an answer for it. Be prepared with a response that reminds you of the commitment you made to yourself. That could be your mantra, or it could just be a quick no-BS check-in with yourself. *How much pain do I really feel? I can catch up on sleep over the weekend. One bite will lead to more, it's just not worth it.* Whatever works for you, do it so that you can get your workout finished, stick to your meal plan, and keep your word to yourself.

Just remember this: The chatter is usually fear disguised as something else. How you deal with it is the truth.

FINDING YOUR "WHY"

As we've discussed, finding your *why*—your deepest motivation for getting healthy—is one of the most important parts of this journey. Knowing your *why* and becoming connected to it will help you hold on to your mantras, quiet the negative chatter, and stay the course.

Getting to this point can be difficult for some people. As a culture and a society, we're just accustomed to the idea of going to the gym or trying to eat right or trying to look better as things we "should" do. These things don't really have any meaning until *we* consciously attach meaning to them.

So what's your story? What do you want to achieve? What has brought you to this point?

And don't go superficial with these answers, either. Dig deep. Let yourself think beyond the *skinny jeans*, the *biceps*, and the *six-pack*. Think deeply about the reasons behind your decision to live a healthier lifestyle.

> *I want to be healthy and a role model for my family.*
> *I want to feel beautiful in my own body.*
> *I want to be able to run around with my kids.*

These reasons, which are different for each person, can be easily and frequently referenced when the going gets tough. In my case, it was an adolescent desire to be accepted—to finally fit in, to feel good about my-self.

What do you *really* want to get out of this program? The more emo-tionally connected you are to the answer to that question, the easier it will be to push through the challenges of getting into shape and the faster you will see results. *What* you are doing in this program is not as important as *why* you are doing it . . . not by a long shot.

Lasting weight loss, like any lasting positive change, is an inside job. External factors come into play only when the mind and heart are in gear. You have to be emotionally connected to your *why* in order to truly suc-ceed. Sure, you can get a fit body by eating well and exercising, but unless the external actions connect to something deeper, the change won't last. If you follow this program closely, your change won't be just on the outside. Your heart and mind will have been transformed as well.

THE ART OF HABIT FORMING

You've probably heard people say that it takes 21 days to make a habit. That's an oversimplification of a complicated concept that seems to per-sist in the minds (and books) of many. A habit is your ability to repeat an action day in and day out, without thought or hesitation. A great book for understanding how habits are formed and changed is *The Power of Habit* by Charles Duhigg.[8] He studied not only individuals but also large corporations to figure out how habits are made, broken, and changed. In the book, he describes a "habit loop" made up of three things: a trigger, an action, and a response.

Let's say you eat too much when you feel stress at work. Boss didn't like your report, deadlines are getting too tight, layoffs are coming—whatever it is, the stress sends you straight to the Burrito Shack around the corner for a belly-filling, stress-squashing pound of south-of-the-border good-ness. In this case, the trigger was the stress at work, the action was eating, and the response was that you felt better, if even for just a while. Even though you knew you'd feel better for only a few hours, the 1,000-calorie burrito-Armageddon you just endured was worth it (at the time) for that response.

One danger is letting yourself get locked into a cycle of triggers and actions. If, for example, every time you sit in front of the TV at night, you want to find a snack or dessert, watching TV becomes a trigger for the action of eating poorly. If you can learn to avoid these types of triggers that are detrimental to your progress, you will be much better off. You can't ever really eliminate work-related stress and maybe your spouse really loves to spend quality time in front of the tube, but if these things are triggers for nutritional disaster, it's best to try to minimize your exposure to these situations. Repetition builds strength and this is just as applicable to mental training as it is physical training.

Day 1 of this program is probably going to kick your butt. Luckily, it will be new, so your resolve and commitment will be high. But around Day 8, when the new-program euphoria has worn off, you might be tempted to skip your workout. That's an opportunity to press through one of those mental reps. Over time, you will develop a habit where you'll feel weird if you *don't* exercise. It might take more than 21 days, but who cares? As long as you're doing it as often as you can, you're training your brain to *want* to do it more and more. Eventually, it becomes second nature.

20-MINUTE MINDSET IN ACTION

So what does it look like to work on your mindset for a few minutes a day? Well, I promise that you're not just going to sit there with your eyes closed, arbitrarily thinking about "things." On this plan, you will engage your mind actively with various mental reps designed to help you build some mind muscle. I call this "Me Time." This is a daily time for you to focus on you: to notice the changes you're experiencing, to build on your success, to confront your challenges, to strengthen your resolve, and to prepare yourself to have another great day tomorrow.

Over time, these periods of reflection will become instinctual. You'll know exactly what you need to get you where you need to go and to continue developing the mental strength that you will carry with you for the rest of your life. But for the first 20 days, I'll offer you some practical exercises that get you into the habit of making this time valuable and productive.

Some days, I might ask you to simply sit and think about where you are in your journey and visualize where you want to go. Other days, I'll have you revisit your deepest motivations—your "why" —by finding and posting photos around your home or office that can serve as reminders of why you're doing what you're doing. Other days, I'll charge you with developing accountability by sharing your journey with others.

Each day, this little bit of brain training helps you to realign your path, to recharge your efforts, and to restore your focus. This time isn't a throwaway in the context of your day. I would argue that the minutes involved are probably the most important few minutes you will spend all day— because if you can't find ways to keep your promises to yourself, then your journey toward greater health will be a daily struggle. I know that over the course of a busy day, when you have so many different responsibilities to juggle, this will feel like the part of the program that you can skip. But I urge you not to skip it. Try to find a way to unplug, to set down your cell, and to turn off the TV and work on this.

A little "Me Time" is just the boost you need to keep going strong over the course of this program. In Chapter 10, we'll take a closer look at these exercises.

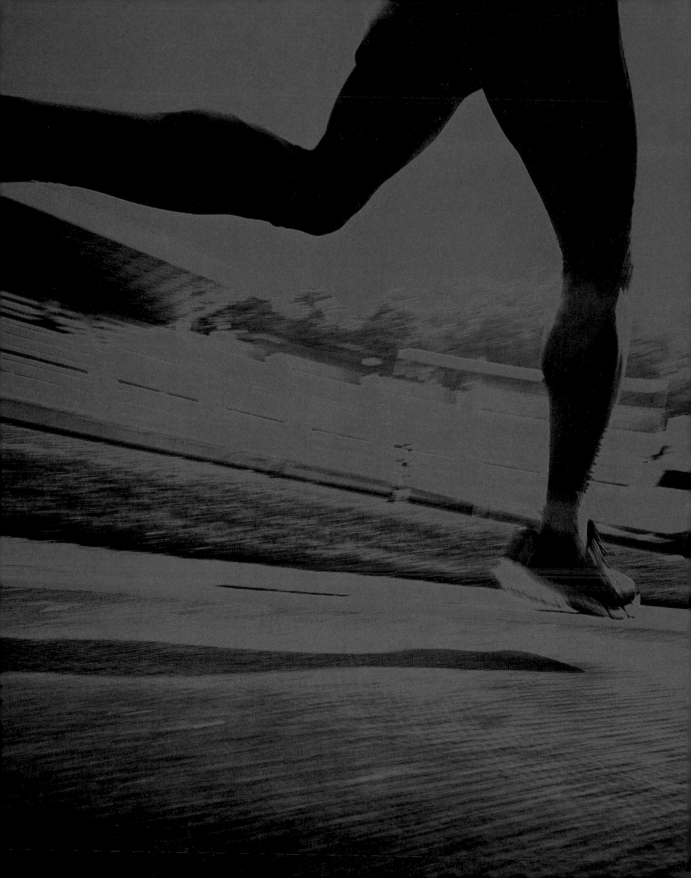

SIX

The Magic of the Afterburn

HOW TO BURN CALORIES WHEN YOU'RE NOT WORKING OUT

B Y NOW, YOU'RE PICKING UP on a central theme: time is precious. I'm so accustomed to working with busy professionals that more condensed, results-oriented training has become second nature to me as a trainer. Shorter workouts help you constantly redefine the limits of what you think your body can do because you really have to dig deep and work hard. But the greatest allure of high intensity training, for many, is how little time it takes. It's a low-cost investment for a high-yield return. It's also the part that critics and skeptics like to criticize.

There's no way you can get anything substantial done in 20 minutes, they'll say. Look, I get it, "longer = better" has been the norm for so long, right? Forty-five minutes to an hour is what most people have come to expect for their training time. But as we discussed in Chapter 3, that formula doesn't seem to be effective for many people. So when some up-start starts singing the praises of a 20-minute workout, it's easy to see how the old guard would take issue.

But the 20-minute scenario is no fad; it is backed by scientific research coupled with my own personal experience with clients and my own train-ing. I have serious doubts that anyone needs to train for 90 minutes to see results. In fact, by going harder for a shorter amount of time, you can burn fat and melt away calories long after your workout is over—trademarks of a body loaded with metabolic muscle.

Another thing that skeptics won't acknowledge is that the *20-Minute Body* is basically the last phase in a fitness evolution that's been in the works for decades. In the '60s, "health culture" took hold, with body-building icons such as Arnold Schwarzenegger and Jack LaLanne com-ing to prominence. In the mid-'90s, functional training with equipment such as BOSU balls, balance boards, and Swiss balls was all the rage. But now, many trainers are advocating shorter, more challenging workouts, and scientists are validating this idea with new studies every day. You see, while my training methods are fresh and fun, the concept of training with greater intensity for less time has been around for quite some time. The more we learn about the human body, the more we are discovering that it is amazingly adaptable. When confronted with something that is a seemingly impossible physical challenge, it just steps up to the plate and adapts. Muscle gets stronger. Lungs use oxygen more efficiently. Body fat starts finding it harder to hold on. And you can get all of those results without spending an hour or more in the gym every day.

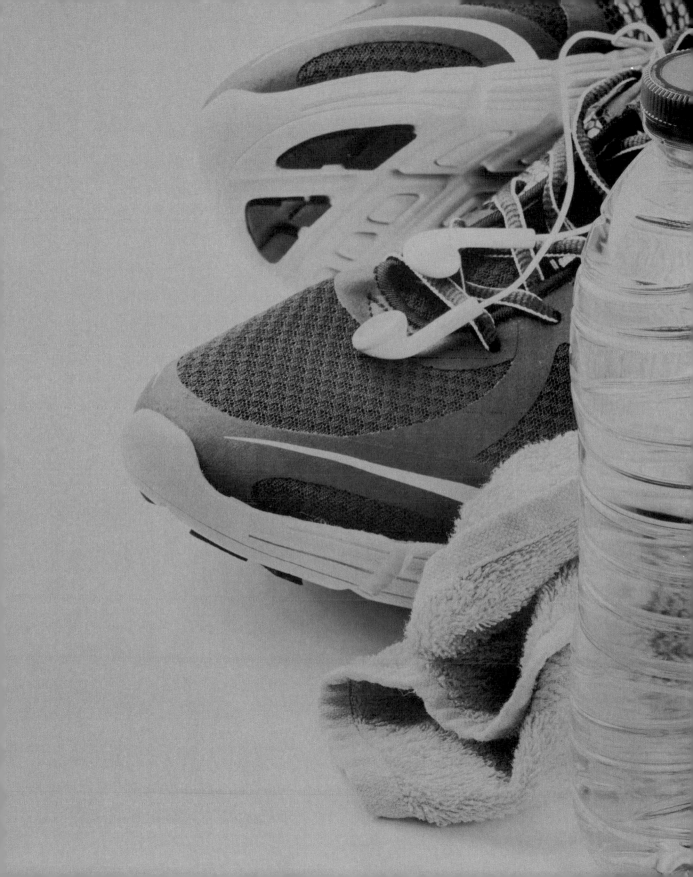

THE SCIENCE OF THE AFTERBURN

Not only do short, intense workouts prevent you from wasting time, but they also help you develop a functional, very athletic physique because they help you develop and strengthen metabolic muscle. That's something you just can't get from training slow all the time. Think about how marathoners look—what they do is amazing but they carry very little muscle and can even look a little flabby. So unless you're going to log 26.2 miles today, chances are that's not the look you're going for.

Let's think about it practically with a real-world example. The mile run is something most people have done at one time or another. It's a tough test sustaining a good pace for that distance. But what if you could sprint your hardest for 100 meters, 16 times, with a little bit of rest after each sprint, then put all those times together for your mile time? (1 mile = 1,600 meters).

The result would be a record-breaking performance because those all-out bursts of intensity, though more physically demanding, are more digestible blocks of work for your body and your mind. And in addition to your new mile mark, you'd have a jacked-up metabolism to boot. This is a prime example of HIIT. And excess post-exercise oxygen consumption, or EPOC (see page 13) is the magical post-workout, fat-fighting party it ignites. I know EPOC may sound like a mythical, too-good-to-be-true phenomenon, but I promise you it is very real.

In fact, one study from the University of Western Ontario (London, Ontario)[9] found that people who ran four to six 30-second sprints with 4 minutes of rest between sprints burned *double* the amount of body fat compared with a group that ran 30–60 minutes at a steady pace. The sprinting group was getting leaner and stronger, with workouts that took less time.

One of the earliest studies in the '90s by researchers at Laval University (Ste-Foy, Quebec, Canada)[10] found that a sprinting group also burned more body fat than a steady-state cardio group . . . despite burning 15,000 calories less. Another head-to-head comparison in an eight-week study at East Tennessee State University in 2001[11] showed that the high intensity interval group dropped 2 percent body fat while the steady runners lost no body fat. And finally, a recent Australian study[12] found that females who did a 20-minute HIIT program lost six times more body fat than a peer group that did a 40-minute cardio routine.

BONUS BENEFITS

As you can see, there are way more benefits to a 20-minute workout than you'd have ever imagined. Well, here's another: it can also help you look and feel younger. Naturally produced growth hormone (GH) is something of a miracle elixir. It does everything from boosting your body's fat burning ability to reducing the effects of aging on your body. Sounds awesome, right? Well, high intensity intervals can help you increase how much of this stuff your body produces by up to 450 percent in the 24 hours after a workout.[13]

And for those of you who like to go for the occasional long run to clear your mind, you can take comfort in knowing that a 20-minute focus isn't going to impede your endurance. In fact, when endurance groups have been pitted head-to-head against sprinting groups, the increases in stamina are similar. And in several studies, interval training groups gained or maintained muscle, which is good for you because it means you can be confident that weight lost is coming from fat, not muscle.

EPOC BEYOND HIIT

In most studies of EPOC, the research focuses on cardio-based interval training. But resistance training also offers a host of benefits. For those of you who are not keen on using weights, just know that resistance includes weights, bands, other tools, and good old-fashioned bodyweight. As long as your muscles are working to overcome (resist) an outside force, you're doing resistance training.

In the next 20 days, you're going to learn a lot of different resistance-based exercises—some will be more dynamic, like striders; and some will be more one-dimensional, like push-ups. Some will be weight-based; others will just be you versus gravity. In every workout, you'll be working major muscle groups with very little time for rest in between sets. And this is where we amplify those EPOC benefits.

While you're training with interval-style protocols—working for 1 minute and resting for 1 minute, for example—the use of resistance with relatively shorter rest is what really jacks up your burn. Research published in *Medicine and Science in Sport and Exercise*[14] found that when subjects lifted with a weight they could handle for up to six repetitions on the leg press, their resting metabolism was elevated for 48 hours after they were done training. And a study out of the College of New Jersey (Ewing)[15] found that when subjects used a weight they could handle for only five reps on the bench press with only 30 seconds of rest between sets, they burned more calories after the workout than a group who trained lighter (10 reps) and with longer rest (3 minutes). Adding structured resistance training to your program—one that targets major muscle groups, challenges them with progressively tougher variations, and relies on little to no rest—can dramatically increase your rate of EPOC. I'll say it again: nothing beats metabolic muscle!

Your body thrives on challenge. The harder you push, the more aggressively it responds by shedding fat and building muscle. Harder exercise, even if we're just talking about cardio, is harder on your body—it gets beaten up and broken down. That sounds bad, I know. Why would we want to beat ourselves up? Because it's all about recovery, that's why. It sounds strange, but when you exercise, you're actually creating microscopic tears in your muscles known as "microtrauma." And guess what? It takes energy to repair those tears, which means that your body needs an energy source, i.e., stored calories. This is why EPOC spikes after exercise done at higher intensities. One study[16] puts the daily amount of additional calories burned per day at 200-plus when you are doing just 2.5 minutes—five 30-second sprints on an exercise bike, each followed by 4 minutes of rest—of interval-style training!

If you've been doing long, monotonous sessions of cardio, you're holding yourself back from your potential. More resistance, less rest, greater intensity . . . it's time to embrace the challenge and benefit of the afterburn.

THE CASE FOR WEIGHTS

Weights are not just for meatheads! No matter what your gender, age, or experience level may be, working out with weights can help change your body. Resistance training also offers a host of health benefits, including:

Improved bone density
Increased metabolism
Improved mobility and balance
Increased release of growth hormone
Improved joint health

BURN BY NUMBERS

2—Percentage of body fat lost in eight weeks of doing interval training.

6X—The amount of body fat lost by an interval-training group when compared with a slow cardio group.

200—Estimated number of additional calories burned per day as a result of 2.5 minutes of interval training.[17]

450—Percent increase in human growth hormone (HGH) in the 24 hours after a high-intensity interval workout.[18]

20-MINUTE FITNESS IN ACTION

You want to be burning calories all the time, whether you're training or not. You want to be full of streamlined, metabolic muscle, ready to tackle any task at hand at a moment's notice. Starting on page 135, I'm going to give you 20 straight days of workouts designed to help you do exactly that. You'll do functional strength and cardio strength workouts to get fitter and then you'll really hit the afterburn with your HIIT workouts when you're ready for them. And when you do those HIIT workouts, you'll definitely know what "HIIT" you—five exercises that use just your bodyweight but will definitely challenge you in new ways.

Since no two people's bodies are the same, I have included three different levels of programs so that you can start in exactly the right place for your age, condition, and fitness level. These workouts will be challenging but also fun and easy to learn so that you can maximize your metabolic muscle over the next 20 days. And once the moves and workouts start feeling too easy, you can do a more advanced version of each exercise or graduate to the next level.

This may be a 20-day program, but it should really be viewed as merely the first phase of your journey to a high-performance body.

HOW INTENSE IS INTENSE?

We talk a lot in this book about intensity and training hard, but what does that mean, exactly? Well, scientists have all sorts of fancy percentages and biomechanical measures to estimate the intensity of physical activity, but for our purposes, the rate of perceived exertion (RPE) will work just fine. This scale, of which there are a few different versions, is a simple way to understand just how hard you're working. Most times, you'll want to be training at the high end of this scale— the higher the number, the higher the afterburn!

RATE OF PERCEIVED EXERTION SCALE

RPE	DESCRIPTION
1	Very light: a pace you can sustain all day while speaking normally
2–3	Light: a slight uptick in heart rate that doesn't impair conversation
4–5	Moderate: starting to get harder, breaking a sweat, speaking a bit labored
6–7	Vigorous: slightly uncomfortable effort, very short of breath
8–9	Very Hard: difficult to maintain your pace or intensity, can speak in short sentences
10	Max Effort: top end of exertion, cannot maintain conversation at all

As you might imagine, your "10" is probably different from your friend's or your workout partner's "10." Don't focus on anyone but yourself, and be honest with your estimates. Remember, your body can always do more than you think it can do.

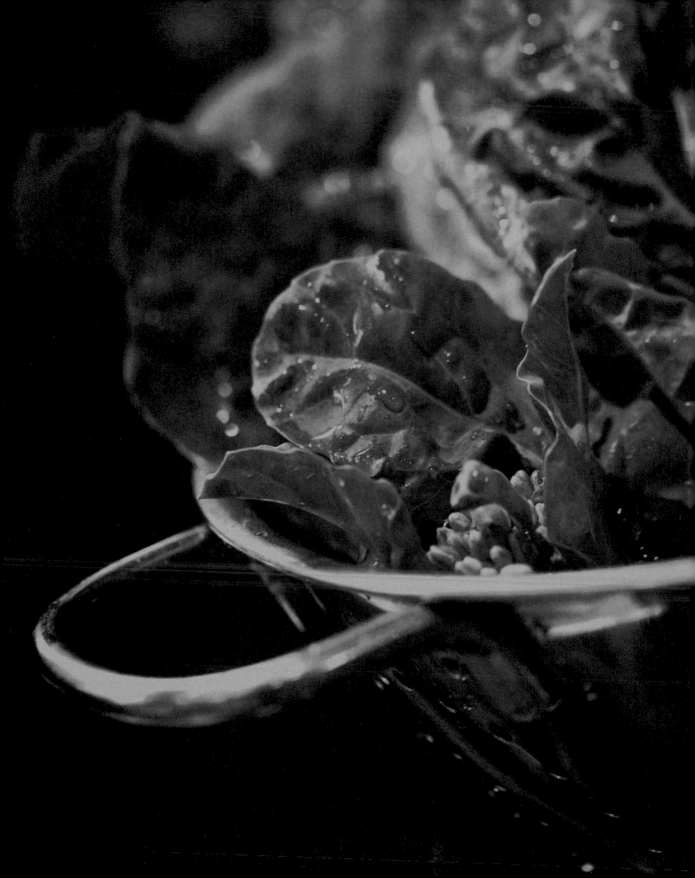

SEVEN

The 20-Minute Diet

GO LEAN, GO GREEN, AND GO CLEAN

NOW THAT YOU have a firm understanding of the brain- and body-training aspects of *The 20-Minute Body*, it's time to get into the part of the formula that will have the greatest impact on what you see in the mirror: nutrition. Exercise creates the stimulus for change, and mindset training helps you stay consistent, but the nutrition is what gives you the fuel to do it all. When you get your nutrition right, you will really see the results you're looking for, like looser-fitting clothes and a noticeably slimmer physique.

This also happens to be the part that trips up most people. I've had plenty of clients over the years who train with me like a beast session after session but after a while we stop seeing results. When I notice stalls like this, I don't ask the clients to train harder or switch up their program. I ask them what they're eating. And 99 percent of the time, they're making mistakes in one or more key areas of their diet. Once we address those problems, the inches and pounds start coming off again.

If you've ever been in that kind of rut—the kind where you're spinning your wheels and getting nowhere with your goals—it's likely to be due to a nutritional issue. You're eating too much or not enough. You're taking in foods that you think are good for you, but they're actually causing you to retain water and bloat. You're not paying attention to how you're eating, when you're eating, or how much variety you include in your diet.

Ironically, those who are the most desperate to lose weight are often the ones who struggle most, because they are more prone to latch on to the latest "diet." And most diets are not nutritionally balanced and are either so restrictive or so tough to follow that people tend to fall off the wagon and often gain even more weight. I've seen it. I've lived it. And for years, I've been helping clients get their nutritional houses in order, not by barraging them with the latest diet information but by *simplifying* things. Because when you make things too complicated, you lose people. Period.

I say toss the scales and the complicated equations and cling to a few basic, easy-to-remember nutritional truths that will make losing inches a cinch. I've broken this down into a no-fuss philosophy: *ditch the white stuff, up the protein, and go lean, green, and clean.*

When you put all five of these tenets to work for you at the same time, you will feel better, you'll have more energy, your workouts will be amazing, and your body will respond to it all by rewarding you with a slimmer, trimmer reflection in the mirror.

DITCHING THE WHITE STUFF

We've already discussed the different types of carbohydrates, and why slow-fueling carbs are generally a better choice than fast-fueling carbs. All of the white, starchy foods that are a staple of our diet in this country, such as white bread, white flour products (crackers, cookies, cakes, etc.), white rice and white rice products (like rice cakes or crackers), and white potatoes (as well as products containing potato starch,) are fast-burning carbs that cause your insulin level to spike when consumed. And remember, your rise in insulin signals your body to store fat. That's definitely not what we want.

Additionally, most of these foods are loaded with nearly unpronounceable lab-generated ingredients, fillers, and other artificial wild cards. You have probably already heard the advice that it's wisest to shop in the outer aisles of the supermarket, where all the perishables are. Fruit, vegetables, nuts, dairy, meats—these are things that are pretty darn close to their natural state and the easiest for your body to process and use for fuel. The majority of the foods that lurk on the shelves of the inside aisles are packaged in bags and boxes and probably went through multiple stages of processing before reaching your store. Loaded with preservatives, these foods are designed to have a long shelf life even though some may be cutting yours short! It's on these shelves that you'll also find many of the fast carbs that we've been talking about. There are exceptions, of course, but most packaged foods are bound to be laden with carbs that provide a quick jolt of energy before sinking you into nap-time mode and taking up permanent residence on your waist and thighs.

But it's easy to enjoy these products without the blood sugar–spiking side effects—just look for the whole, unprocessed versions that have kept the fiber intact. This ensures that you still get to enjoy these foods, if just in slightly different, healthier-for-you forms. Go for brown rice and whole wheat flour or other whole grain or nut-based flours, and enjoy sweet potatoes instead of white potatoes. Sweet potatoes don't affect your blood sugar or insulin in the same way as white potatoes—they're full of slow-burning carbs and digestion-slowing fiber that make them a superior choice most of the time.

But there are a few more white foods that are hurting you that aren't as widely addressed as refined carbs: namely, salt, sugar, and milk.

Salt and sugar are two of the most problematic because they are hidden *everywhere* in our diet. Most processed foods contain high levels of salt and sugar, which light up our taste buds and keep us coming back for more. Salt is also a preservative, meaning that it helps to keep processed foods shelf-stable so they can sit in grocery stores and be sellable longer. Even when you are trying to avoid them, added salt and sugar often appear in places you wouldn't expect, like "health" bars and powders, beef jerky, tomato sauce, cereal, yogurt, and other items. It can sometimes feel as if these "white devils" are stalking you, finding new and creative ways to infiltrate your diet and derail your fat loss.

By itself, salt isn't a bad thing. We need a certain amount of sodium in our bodies to power the heart and other muscular functions. Sodium is required to keep nerves and muscles functioning optimally and communicating with the brain. These are good things! I'm not an advocate of calorie-counting so I'm certainly not going to ask you to count sodium milligrams, but it does help to know the recommended daily allowance so you can factor it into your meals. Most organizations, from the American Heart Association (AHA) to the United States Department of Agriculture (USDA), recommend consuming no more than 1,500–2,300 mg per day. Sounds like a lot, right? But consider that one serving of canned chicken soup can contain upwards of 340 mg sodium, and you can start to see how quickly that allowance adds up if you aren't careful.

Too much sodium can have serious consequences for your health. One of the less serious but most immediate and noticeable effects is *bloating*. Foods with excess salt cause water retention beneath the skin, giving you a "puffy" or "doughy" appearance, even if you're generally lean. It's your body's way of restoring balance. As sodium levels rise, your body holds on to more water in order to dilute the sodium. This can be mitigated through additional water consumption (which excretes sodium through urine) or activity (which excretes sodium through sweat). You've probably experienced the effects of a salt overdose firsthand. One dinner with a bit too much soy sauce and you could wake up looking 10 pounds heavier in the mirror. This is particularly true of women, who are sometimes more susceptible to bloating than men, owing to hormonal changes that occur around menstrual cycles. In short, we are probably all having way too much sodium each day.

To optimize the health benefits, you want to try to keep within the specified ranges by avoiding foods that carry excessive amounts of salt.

Sugar is probably the most widely known waistline-widening substance on the planet, but it is still consumed in epic amounts by Americans. In 1822, most Americans averaged 45 grams of sugar over the course of five days. In 2012, that number has skyrocketed to 765 grams of sugar in the same time frame. It's estimated that Americans consume 3,550 pounds of sugar over a lifetime.[19] The problem is partly lack of awareness, partly lack of discipline. Most of us aren't aware of just how much sugar we're putting away every day. But once we do know, we should be shocked into action.

SALT & SUGAR LIMITS

You should **avoid** foods with more than **100 mg of sodium.**
You should **avoid** foods with more than **10 g of sugar**, unless it has 5 g or more of fiber.

Consumed sugar causes fat storage by increasing your body's release of insulin. That release of insulin causes your body to retain sodium, which causes you to retain more water. It's an ugly cycle! But the effects of sugar are more dire than what the mirror might reflect. Those insulin spikes from processed and/or fast-digesting sugars not only have a terrible impact on our weight, body composition, and joints but can also contribute to inflammation, arthritis, diabetes, premature aging, and depressed immunity.[20] A recent study published in the *JAMA Internal Medicine* found that those who consumed 15 percent of their daily calories from sugar were 18 percent more likely to die from cardiovascular disease. And for those who consumed over 21 percent, their risk of death from cardiovascular disease doubled. This correlation was found to exist pretty much across the board in the test group—risk didn't vary depending on gender, weight, physical activity, or even smoking! Sugar increases blood pressure, raises levels of bad cholesterol while decreasing levels of good cholesterol, and may enhance the genetic effects of obesity.

We like to think of sugar as it relates to our ability to keep body fat low but as the science shows, it can literally be a life-and-death issue. When it comes to salt and sugar, we're overdoing it. Because they are hidden in so many of the foods that make up our usual diets, we end up eating more of them than we realize and certainly more than we would if we were more aware of what excess amounts can do to the body. We're conditioned to favor—in fact, *crave*—foods that have been flavored with these ingredients, and food manufacturers know it. People who have tried to go low sugar or low sodium know: after just a day or two, your body aches for foods that contain those things and, unless you are a pillar of willpower, it's hard not to give in.

Another white food I urge people to avoid is cow's milk. I know I know . . . it's supposed to "do a body good." And it can. Milk is a good source of protein, calcium, and vitamin D, but there are many health concerns regarding this table staple that many people aren't even aware of. In fact, a great many people suffer health issues strictly as a result of consuming milk and they don't even realize it.

Part of the problem is that many people are lactose intolerant. They lack enough of an enzyme called lactase to break it down for use by the body and the result is cramping, bloating, gas, diarrhea, and colon irritation. Also, many of today's dairy cows are fed rBGH, or recombinant growth hormone, which helps them produce more milk by increasing their levels of IGF-1 (insulin-like growth factor-1). Unfortunately, many of these cows suffer more udder infections, which means they are fed more antibiotics, which are then passed on to the end consumer. The effect of this process on humans is of some debate in the scientific community but as a consumer, you have the right—and perhaps the responsibility—to choose foods that are closest to their most natural state. You just want the milk. You're not signing up for rBGH and IGF-1 and all the other nonsense.

Luckily, dairy isn't the only game in town—alternatives like almond, rice, coconut, and soy milk are pleasing to the palate and have none of the unwanted side effects of dairy milk. Protein-rich soy comes with an asterisk, as well, as it may increase estrogen production and many brands have also been treated with chemicals to increase production.

Understanding that many people out there still consume cow's milk,

I'm simply urging a *gradual* shift away from it. You can start my program on organic skim milk, which is lower in calories and fat, but as you move through the program, we'll move to alternative milk choices, eventually leaving cow's milk behind altogether. Unsweetened coconut, almond, soy, and rice milk are strong choices, too. And if you are able to pivot away from cow's milk completely, I doubt you'll even miss it.

GOING LEAN, CLEAN, AND GREEN

Eliminating these white foods from your diet is the first step in getting your nutrition in check. Just by doing that, you're helping your body detox and become more efficient at burning fat, shedding water, and converting energy. Once you make the swaps (see sidebar) that I'm suggesting, you'll be taking in far more nutritious foods, cutting calories, and giving your body a break from riding the insulin roller coaster. You will notice a difference within days.

The next step in going lean, clean, and green is to fill your diet with lean sources of protein, clean unprocessed foods, and lots of green (and other brightly colored) vegetables.

GO LEAN

Protein helps produce valuable molecules in the body such as enzymes and hormones that keep our immune system, muscles, organs, and brain working in top condition. But its greatest benefit may be that it is the building block of all muscle. It contains amino acids that are critical for rebuilding muscle, which, as you learned in Chapter 1, keeps you strong and metabolic since muscle burns more calories than fat. Protein truly is the wonder macronutrient, because there is practically no downside to it. It digests slowly, helps to rebuild muscle tissue (after injury or from training), keeps you feeling fuller for longer, and is an important building block for skin, hair, bones, and blood.

Yes, I know, sweeteners and dairy are two of your favorite things. Even the healthiest among us consume a lot of milk and sugar on a daily basis. And in the absence of sugar, many people turn to artificial sweeteners. I want you to clean up your sweetener habit because these chemicals have very little upside when it comes to losing weight and maintaining health. My 20-day nutrition plans will walk you through some gradual changes that you can make, but if you want to start trying some of these things early, here's a list of picks that are both tasty and good for you!

MILK SWAPS	BRETT SAYS . . .
Almond Milk	Full of vitamin E and calcium and very low in calories (40 per 8-ounce serving), the unsweetened version is great for baking, quiches, cereals, and puddings. Unsweetened vanilla almond is still sweet, just with fewer calories.
Coconut Milk	Higher in energy-producing vitamin B_3 (and calories) than dairy milk, coconut milk is a great cooking substitute for milk or cream and can be used in quiches, pies, puddings, and custards, and cold on cereal. It can be a bit thick so you may want to try it thinned out with a bit of other nondairy milk. If you're a coffee drinker, coconut creamers are a strong choice because they look and taste like real cream!
Rice Milk	Rice milk is cholesterol-free, contains no lactose, and is lower in fat and calories than whole milk. It can be on the sweet side, but

Rice Milk (con't)	·········	it's easy to digest for many people and a good replacement for hot or cold cereal and in smoothies and other beverages.
Goat's Milk	········· →	Goat's milk yogurts and cheeses are good because they are more fermented than the cow's milk versions and contain more enzymes that allow you to digest the milk protein. The problem for many people is that sour taste. Try a natural sweetener to taste if that's the case.

SWEETENER SWAPS		BRETT SAYS . . .
Stevia	········· →	Stevia is a plant-based sweetener that suppresses cravings and contains zero calories, and since it's so potent, you need only a little.
Honey	········· →	Honey is absorbed by the body more slowly than table sugar, so it has less impact on blood sugar; and since it is also sweeter, you generally need less of it.
Maple Syrup	········· →	With more body-friendly potassium and calcium, and fewer carbs, maple syrup can help to sweeten a number of dishes in place of traditional sugar. But since it is still high in carbs from sugar, intake should still be kept modest.
Coconut Sugar	········· →	It contains about the same amount of calories as regular sugar, but it's full of fiber, iron, zinc, and potassium, making it the winner in a head-on competition.

It takes a lot of work for your body to digest, absorb, and use protein—much more than it takes for carbs or fat. This is great when protein is digested by itself and even better when you pair protein with foods like carbs and healthy fats, as it slows the process to a crawl. This greatly reduces the impact on your blood sugar, which is what you want in order to minimize the chances that food will be stored as fat. This also gives you a steady, consistent stream of energy and keeps you fuller longer. It's a craving crusher!

And when you're doing strength training, it's crucial to get enough protein, because when you break down muscle tissue through progressively tougher training, your muscles are open and starving to be fed amino acids. I suggest eating a little bit of protein at every meal and around workouts to ensure that you are properly feeding your muscles.

But here's the key: we are talking about lean proteins—turkey, chicken breast, lean beef and pork, fish and tofu. Yes, this means you'll have to ditch your wings, double cheeseburgers, and cheese steaks. Don't worry, though. I'm going to teach you how to pick the leanest proteins and how to cook them in a way that is bursting with flavor.

GO CLEAN

When I talk about "clean" foods, I mean foods that are in their most natural state, not processed or refined in any way. If it comes in a box, a bag, or a cellophane wrapper, it's probably not clean. And if you *have to* buy prepared foods, read labels carefully. Stay away from foods with ingredients you can't pronounce (they're mostly chemicals) as well as those with long ingredient lists (aim for fewer than five ingredients).

Many processed foods also contain hydrogenated fats and synthetic sugars. Steer clear of anything that lists hydrogenated oils or high fructose corn syrup on the label. Hydrogenated oils, a processed version of naturally occurring oils, have been linked to chronic disease and can interfere with blood pressure. And because of the composition of high fructose corn syrup—a widely used form of processed sugar, which consists of glucose and fructose—it is digested much faster by the body and can result in staggering spikes in fat-storing insulin.

And be very cautious of "diet" foods that advertise themselves as "fat free" or "sugar free." The fat-free stuff is loaded with salt, sugar, and chemicals, and the sugar-free stuff usually contains sucralose, aspartame, or another synthetic sweetener. There are no Splenda trees or NutraSweet plants in nature. The body does not recognize these substances as food and they have no nutritive value. Though early reports on artificial sweeteners like saccharin showed a link to cancer, more modern analysis by the Mayo Clinic[22] has largely disproved that. But researchers at Harvard urge a more cautious approach to artificial sweeteners because they can cause us to crave more sugars, which can lead to overconsumption of calories, which can lead to weight gain, which can lead to a host of other maladies[23] including metabolic syndrome and diabetes. Better options include natural fats like coconut or olive oil and natural sweeteners like stevia, honey, agave, or maple syrup.

THE GMO DEBATE

One of the most oft-discussed but little understood acronyms in the health food world is GMO. Genetically modified organisms are organisms whose genetic materials have been altered by means of genetic engineering techniques. That sounds overwhelming . . . because it is. But for you, as a consumer, it is good enough to know that scientists are creating hybrids of plants and animals that are more resistant to disease and may be grown or bred to promote specific beneficial traits. More food to the market sounds like a good thing but the problem is that little is understood about what effect these foods may have on humans.

In keeping with our philosophy of eating foods as close as possible to their natural state, I'd recommend steering clear of GMOs *when possible*—more and more companies are beginning to label their foods as "non-GMO." But until GMO/non-GMO labeling is required of all companies, you would do well to simply buy foods labeled "organic," which are produced through old-fashioned, organic farming.

Our nutrition is going to focus on clean foods like vegetables, simple grains, lean proteins, healthy fats, and fruit. I like to say that if a food existed on the planet 1,000 years ago, there's a good chance that it's really healthy for you. Going "clean" is kind of a no-brainer dietary approach because you can know exactly what you're putting in your body—there's no guesswork or calorie counting, because you will be eating nutritious, fiber-rich foods that are difficult to overeat. And I'm easy on you at first—you will gradually detox from the bad stuff until you are eating only the good stuff. By shifting *gradually* to a healthier way of eating, you won't "shock" your body and you'll get used to new foods and new ways of preparing them in a way that becomes automatic and enjoyable.

GO GREEN

Like most of us, you probably spent your childhood fighting your mom about eating spinach and broccoli. Because of all these early battles at the dinner table, you might be left with a little post-traumatic stress about getting your greens. But folks, Popeye (and your mom) had it right, there's power in spinach.

Greens have absolutely no downside. They're affordable, packed with fiber, and nearly calorie-free. But calorie-free doesn't mean nutrient-free. Green veggies are loaded with vitamins that your body needs to keep working efficiently. Vitamins A and C, for example, are abundant in kale, turnip greens, Swiss chard, spinach, and broccoli. Vitamin A helps with vision and cell growth, while vitamin C is the undisputed king of immune system function. Other veggies such as peas, cucumbers, and celery are rich in lutein, which is good for your eyes. Collectively, green veggies have been shown to reduce your risk of heart attack and stroke,[24] and this may be part of the reason that green foods and juices are so popular now. Yesterday's veggie-shunning generations are today's health food store shoppers!

Guess what else? Because of their high fiber content, veggies slow down digestion and they are *filling*! This means that you are far less likely to go foraging through your fridge or break for the vending machine if you've had your greens.

And since I don't recommend traditional cow's milk, you might be wondering where you're going to make up for all the calcium you'll be missing. The answer is also the produce aisle. To continue getting enough of this bone-, nerve- and muscle-boosting mineral, make sure you pick up collard greens, kale, turnip greens, and arugula, which are all high in calcium.

Going "green" is great but you are welcome to branch out to other colors when it comes to your vegetables. Ideally, try to create a rainbow on your plate—choose brightly colored veggies like bell peppers, beets, and eggplant, which tend to contain more cell-safeguarding antioxidants.

So yes . . . greens and other veggies will be an important part of how you eat on the *20-Minute Body* plan. You'll feel better while reducing overall calorie intake and—this may be the best part—your mom will be proud of you!

20-MINUTE NUTRITION IN ACTION

You're cutting out the white stuff and eliminating processed foods that are making it hard for you to get healthier and leaner, foods that are robbing you of energy and plundering your metabolism. Instead, you're going lean, clean, and green to give your body the highest-quality fuel possible, which will power your workouts and your health.

Yes, you have to cook, which takes a little bit of time, but I promise you're going to be in the kitchen for 20 minutes or less. You will be amazed at how simple it is to eat healthfully and how much great food you can make in a short period of time. With some tips on food preparation, batch cooking methods, and a ton of flavoring options, you will never get bored and you'll never spend too much time in the kitchen. My promise to you is that I'll teach you how to take the meals you already love and are already cooking for your family, and make them healthier, tastier, *and faster to prepare*. I'll show you how to seamlessly phase in cleaner options over time so that you can consistently eat in a way that supports metabolic muscle and keeps you burning fat around the clock.

GREEN GUIDE

Once you go green, it'll be easy to go lean. Here are some of the top nutrient-dense picks you can make when selecting green veggies.

VEGGIE	PERK
Kale	This generation's broccoli, kale is much maligned for its "earthy" taste, but once you learn how to cook with it, you won't look back. This leafy green is packed, gram for gram, with more bone-boosting calcium than milk (125 vs. 100 for milk). It is also rich in magnesium, which plays a huge part in blood pressure regulation and heart function, as well as vitamins A, C, K, and B_6.
Collards	A staple in Southern dishes, collards can definitely be added to a great many more family menus. They're calorie-light (46 per 100 g) and are highly touted for their abundance of cancer-fighting compounds such as diindolylmethane and sulforaphane.

VEGGIE	PERK
Spinach	Vitamins A and C for immunity, iron for healthy blood and improved energy. Yeah. Spinach has you covered on that stuff. But it also contains more blood-and-bone–boosting vitamin K per cup than nearly every other vegetable.
Broccoli	Don't skip the broccoli on your dinner plate. It is famous not only for the fear it strikes into children's hearts but for its myriad health benefits including its many links to the prevention of several different kinds of cancer. A new study indicates that this superfood may even help to fight air pollution in your lungs![25] Broccoli also has high levels of vitamin K and has been shown to help lower cholesterol.

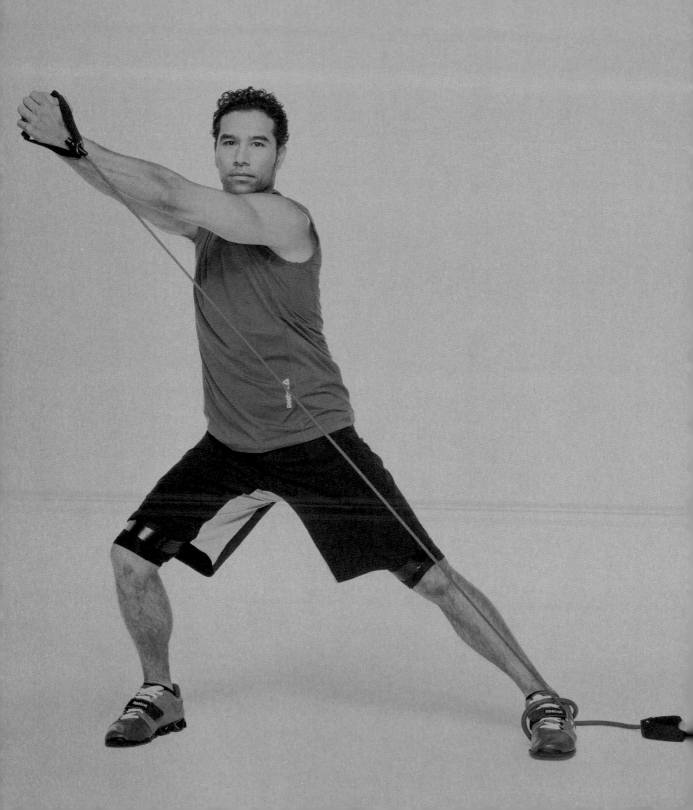

EIGHT

Yellow, Orange, and Blue

SET YOURSELF UP FOR SUCCESS

W E'VE DISCUSSED THE IMPORTANCE of metabolic muscle and explained how we're going to train for it. We outlined how going "lean, clean, and green" sets you up for dietary success and helps you lose inches fast. And we explained how crucial your mindset training is and what it will entail. Each of these things takes only minutes a day but will leave you slimmer, trimmer, healthier, and more energetic than you've felt in years . . . maybe ever.

The journey starts now. Now we're going to look at the three different levels of the *20-Minute Body* fitness plan, and assess your level of fitness right now.

COLOR PROGRESSIONS

From this point forward, you'll notice the insertion of three colors into the mix: yellow, orange, and blue. When I first started training in the

Afro-Brazilian martial art of capoeira ("kap-way-rah"), I loved the whole notion of how students progressed through the ranking system. When you become a capoeira student, you begin a progression of lessons that are expressed in the color of the cord you wear as part of your uniform. It doesn't matter how skilled you are when you walk in the door—everyone starts at white.

That's why I've created color levels in the *20-Minute Body* program. The color levels in my program build, one on another. You'll start with the yellow program, using the progressions I've noted for you to make the exercises harder when you're ready for an additional challenge. After completing the yellow *20-Minute Body* program in 20 days, you'll have the opportunity to do the 20-day orange-level program. And after two 20-day programs, you can graduate to the 20-day blue program. In all, I've given you three 20-day programs so that you can set progressive goals for yourself.

But don't take this progression lightly. It goes beyond the colors. In fitness, we abide by a principle called SAID, which stands for specific adaptations to imposed demands. In a nutshell, the harder you push your body over time at a given activity, the more it is apt to respond. The "imposed demands" of my fitness plan for you are designed to help you build functional, metabolic muscle that keeps you burning fat around the clock. And by gradually turning up the heat, you give your body a chance to adapt.

If you consistently train the same way, with the same weights, using the same exercises and the same rest periods, your body will quickly plateau and refuse to add any more muscle or strength or to shed any more body fat. This is a fact. You have to make gradual progress by adding a bit more weight, condensing rest periods, adding more difficult exercises, and just generally challenging your body to do new things. And when you do, amazing things happen! You find that you are doing things you never thought possible and that your body *will* do what you ask of it. You just have to set the bar higher and higher to make that happen.

The fitness programs here are written with that in mind. From yellow to blue, each exercise included will have easier and more advanced versions that you can implement depending on your skill level. That's great. But the elements of the programming—the actual exercises, sets, reps, and time—are put in place for a specific purpose and one definitely builds on the one before it.

You might feel the temptation to dive into the orange or blue program and I can't stop you from doing that. But I've been doing this a long time and I can tell you that when you do too much, too soon, things become difficult very quickly. In the case of exercise, it can leave you injured, frustrated, and with more fat and inflammation than ever before. Starting at yellow and making the progressions in the correct order is the best way to ensure success.

I've also had clients who have repeated levels and seen different and improved results. For example, if you're a beginner and you run through the yellow level a second time starting on Day 21, you're going to absolutely slay those workouts because you'll be training with more strength and stamina than you had on Day 1. And you'll get more out of those workouts. So don't think that just because yellow is a starting point, it's easy or remedial. I am going to expect 100 percent at every level.

The color level doesn't define you; the work does!

At the beginning of this book, I said that by following this program to the letter, you could lose up to 20 inches from all over, and I meant it. But that will be dependent upon you and how well you keep your promises to yourself. Because when things get complicated or difficult, it's easy to skip a workout, or go digging through the junk drawer for pizza coupons. Preparation is everything. Ben Franklin famously said, "By failing to prepare, you are preparing to fail." And nowhere is that more true than in the areas of health and fitness.

FITNESS PREP: ESTABLISHING YOUR BASELINE

In order to set accurate fitness goals, it's a good idea to test your current level of fitness in a few specific areas. This isn't a way to judge and feel bad about yourself if you're not where you want to be with your fitness. It's just a way to take a baseline assessment that you can test yourself against later to have a definitive, measurable gauge of your progress. I can guarantee that you'll be amazed at how far you've progressed after you complete each level.

So let's get started. Before you do this fitness test, be sure to do a short warm-up (see sidebar). This workout represents square one. Rest at least one day after this baseline assessment before starting Day 1 of the program.

WARMING UP: THE WORK BEFORE THE WORKOUT

If you're working out with me, you're going to have to get used to warming up first. This is the most often overlooked and underrated part of any training program. A good warm-up increases blood flow, wakes up your nervous system, and prepares muscles for the work ahead, fortifying you against injury in the process. There's nothing worse than starting a program fully motivated, only to strain something right out of the gate. Take these steps before any activity to maximize success and minimize risk.

- **TO GET YOUR HEART RATE UP:** Step or jog in place, and do some light jumping jacks or step-outs for 2–3 minutes. You should be breathing harder and your heart rate should be up. In most cases, you'll have a light sweat going.

- **TO OPEN UP YOUR LEGS:** Swing each leg forward and backward, and side to side, while holding on to a chair for balance.

- **TO STRETCH YOUR LEGS:** Perform a quadriceps stretch by holding your ankle with your right hand, keeping your left leg straight, holding on to a chair for balance. (Variation: Kneel on a mat or rug and step your left leg out so that both legs are at 90-degree angles. Grab your right foot with your right hand and gently pull your right heel toward you.) Switch sides. Perform a hamstring stretch by bending your left leg, extending your right leg to the ground so that the heel touches the ground, and hinging down (think of pushing your booty up and away from your hips to activate the back of your legs).

- **TO WARM UP YOUR LOWER LEGS AND FEET:** Rock back and forth on your toes with your knees in a deep squat and hands on the ground to stretch out your toes and feet.

- **TO WARM UP YOUR BACK AND UPPER BODY:** Stand upright with arms out in a T position. Swing to one side and then the other several times. Reach your arms above your head to stretch your shoulders. Cross your arms in front of you and then behind you to open up your upper back.

RUN/WALK TEST | This movement assesses your **aerobic endurance**.

WHAT YOU NEED: An outdoor area where you can run/walk for about 10 minutes (such as a running path).

THE TEST: This test is meant to assess improvements in your aerobic endurance. Choose a set distance that you're comfortable completing by running, jogging, or jogging with a few walking intervals. This can be a quarter mile (or so) for new athletes, a half mile if you've been exercising for a while, or even a mile if you're comfortable at that distance. The distance isn't as important as the length of time you're moving: 2–4 minutes or so for beginners, and up to 9–11 minutes for experienced athletes. Cover your chosen distance and **time the result**.

REST: 1–3 minutes

DISTANCE:_____   **TIME:**_____

PUSH-UP | This movement assesses your **upper-body strength**.

WHAT YOU NEED: An exercise mat or soft floor surface, like a rug.

STARTING POSITION: Start with your body in plank position: hands and toes on the ground supporting your body weight, straight body, with hands placed outside your shoulders.

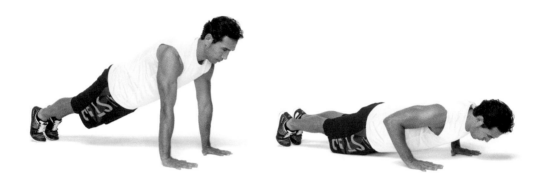

Slowly lower your body, keeping your spine straight, until your chest is just above the ground.

Push back to your starting position.

VARIATION: If this movement feels challenging right now, keep your knees on the ground.

GOAL: Perform as many repetitions as you can, to failure. Your goal is 30 full-body push-ups for men, and 10 for women.

REST: 1 minute

REPS:_____

SQUAT | This movement assesses your **lower-body strength**.

STARTING POSITION: Stand with your feet a little wider than hip distance apart, toes pointing forward. Cross your arms over your chest, with your elbows lifted toward the horizon so that your arms are parallel to the floor.

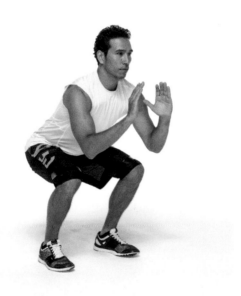

GOAL: Bend both knees to 90 degrees, thighs parallel to the floor, and push through your heels to return to the starting position. Perform as many repetitions as you can, to failure.

REST: 1 minute

REPS:_____

BENT-OVER ROW | This movement assesses your **back and core strength**.

WHAT YOU NEED: Two hand weights (8–10 pounds each), or an exercise band.

STARTING POSITION: Stand with your feet about hip distance apart. Bend forward from your hips so that your upper body is at about a 45-degree angle to the floor. You should have a weight in each hand or an exercise band.

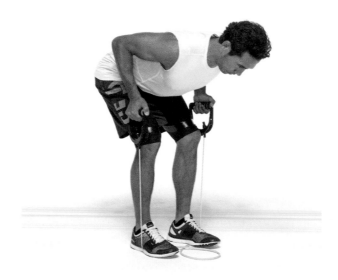

GOAL: Perform as many repetitions as you can, to failure.

REST: 1 minute

REPS:_____

PLANK | This movement assesses your **core strength and endurance**.

STARTING POSITION: Start in a plank position (same as the starting position for the push-up), but with your forearms on the floor.

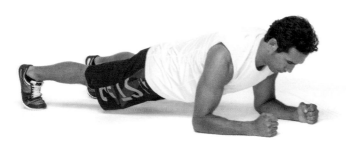

GOAL: Hold this position as long as you can without lowering your knees to the ground. Record the amount of time you can hold the position.

REST: 1 minute

TIME:_____

COBRA | This movement assesses your **core (especially lower back) strength and endurance**.

STARTING POSITION: Lie on the floor (stomach down) with your arms extended. You can have your arms in a "T," a "W," or a "Y" position.

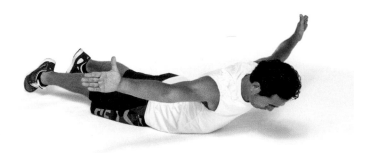

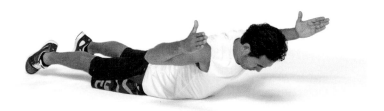

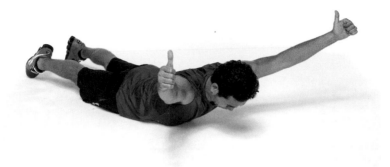

GOAL: Lift your upper body while keeping your lower body and feet on the floor. Hold this position as long as you can. Record the amount of time you can hold the position.

REST: 1 minute

TIME:_____

LOG IT

One workout in the books. You may feel as if you've been put through the meat grinder and that's okay. It's not how you start, it's how you finish. Be accurate and honest with each of these assessments, jotting down your exact performance metrics (reps, time, etc.). What you write down today will serve as a valuable tool for you throughout the program because as you get stronger and build more stamina, these reference points will help you build confidence in how far you've come and in how far you have the potential to go.

This isn't a pass-or-fail test. It's simply a measurable indicator of your starting condition.

WITNESS YOUR FITNESS

Many goals are emotional and mental and may not be easy to track. Through the mindset exercises in Chapter 10, I encourage you to explore these things. But as your trainer for these 20 days, I want to help you come up with the best physical indicators of your progress in a few key areas. In addition to your other journaling efforts, make sure to take note of these tangibles on or ahead of Day 1.

PICTURES

In the workout groups and challenge contests I lead, I find that participants who have really compelling before-and-after photos stay motivated and excited because they can see their progress. By referencing these photos later on, you may find that your clothes are fitting better or that your complexion has started to improve. These photos are every bit as valuable as your daily appointments with the mirror because they provide immediate, visual evidence of how far you've come. To get your before-and-after right, follow these steps:

1. Photos should be full body, head to toe, with a solid wall or background behind you. Stand shoeless with your feet hip width apart.

2. Take two photos from the front: one with your hands at your hips, and the other with your hands at your sides.

3. Take two photos from the right side: one with your hands at your hips, and the other with your hands at your sides. Repeat on your left side.

4. Your clothing should be snug, not baggy. Use the same clothes for each set of photos (for example, on Day 1, Day 10, and Day 20).

MEASUREMENTS

Yes, you can lose 20 inches in 20 days. But what does that look like? Most people are at least mildly familiar with taking a waist measurement, but this is only one of several sites that you will measure to determine the total amount of inches lost. You may lose a few inches from your waistline, sure . . . but the most telling indicator is how many inches you've lost from *everywhere*.

Using a flexible tape measure, you should take your circumference stats at each of the following sites. Ideally, this is done with a partner helping you.

- **BUSTLINE:** With your arms up and out to your sides, like a plane, the tape measure is placed across the nipple line. Once the tape measure is set, place your arms at your sides, inhale, and take the measurement.

- **ARMS:** This is measured on the upper arm, between the top of the shoulder and the elbow, in a relaxed position. Take the measurement for the other arm as well. Don't worry if the readings are different: we aren't symmetrical . . . it's normal!

- **WAIST:** This is taken right across the belly button, tape measure parallel to the floor.

• **HIPS:** Measure around the widest part of the hips/butt. Not everyone loves this one, but it's a great indicator of progress since this is such a problem area for many people.

• **ABDUCTORS:** Measure the upper portion of the thighs just below the glutes. This is a measurement of both thighs, so the tape goes all the way around in the same manner that the waist and hips were measured.

• **THIGHS:** Take a big step to the right and measure the circumference of your thigh about $1^1/_2$ inches down from your inseam, then repeat with the other leg. This area is the largest part of the thigh.

POUNDS

The scale is the least important factor on this program, but it still serves as one of many indicators of how you're doing. People with more weight to lose will probably see the most movement here, but for the most part, you should be focusing on how you look in the mirror and in your photos, what your measurements are, and how you are feeling overall. Weigh yourself no more than once per week.

All of these areas will represent your starting point—the baseline evidence that you can continue to come back to at any time to measure your progress. Don't get into the habit of doing this too frequently. Ideally, you should consult these baseline indicators at the end of each 20-day block.

READY, SET . . .

Part of appreciating the journey is knowing where you started. When it comes to our bodies, it's hard to exercise patience. You start a new program like this one and you want to see change right away. You want to see your waistline thinning, your hips slimming, and your tummy flattening. You want to feel stronger and more energetic and you want all of these things right now. The reality is that it doesn't happen overnight—and also you are not the best judge, because you're too close! Over 20 days, you might not see the day-to-day changes you're experiencing, but those around you might ask, "Hey, are you doing something different?" or "Did you lose some weight?" And if you're still in doubt, these assessments that you've done in this chapter will be proof positive of the work you've put in. I actually encourage my clients to repeat these initial assessments after a few weeks so they can see how far they've come. I promise, if you put in the work, you won't be disappointed!

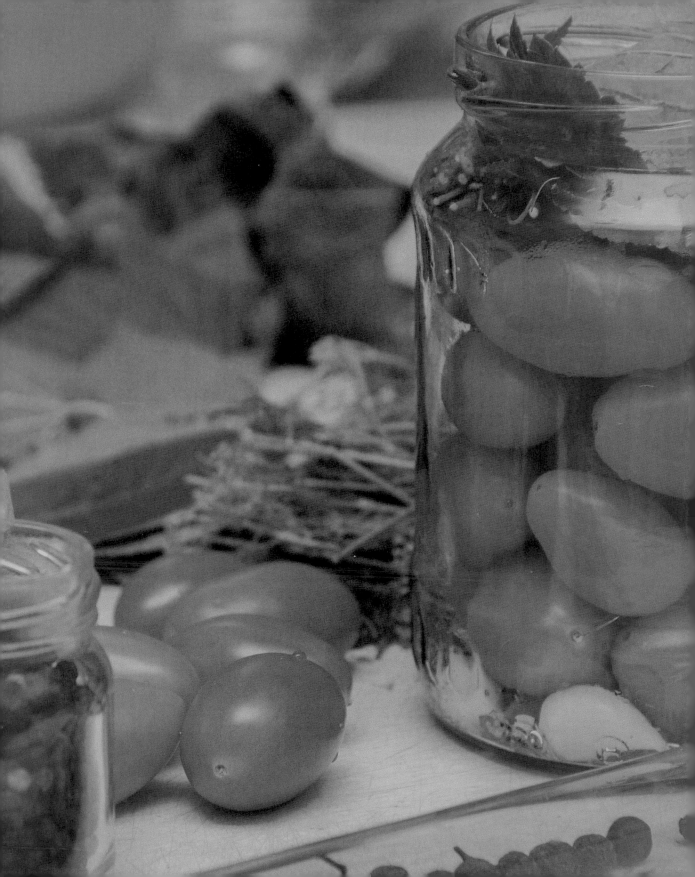

NINE

Kitchen Prep

GETTING READY FOR NUTRITIONAL SUCCESS

THE KITCHEN. This is really where weight loss battles are won and lost. As we outlined in Chapter 7, what you are feeding your body will determine just how much you are able to change your body in the next 20 days and beyond. A lot of what you do with regard to your nutrition will hinge on your motivation, but a lot also depends on how well prepared you are to eat well. When you get set up with the right tools and the right foods, you save time and money while losing pounds and inches.

To help you get your kitchen prepped for dietary dominance, let's go over everything you need, including pantry essentials, spices and herbs that will help you cut down your reliance on sugar and salt for flavor, and the essential kitchen tools that make cooking in 20 minutes a cinch.

But first things first: Get into your pantry and fridge and toss out everything that's past its expiration date and any processed food or "white stuff" that is standing between you and your goal. All set? Good. Time to get serious, people!

NUTRITION FOR YELLOW, ORANGE, AND BLUE

This is a no-deprivation diet. There's no calorie counting and no starving yourself. But in order to go "lean, clean, and green," we're getting rid of as many processed foods as possible and introducing 20 delicious herbs and spices that will become your go-to arsenal of flavor. We're also going to work on getting rid of the white stuff in your diet—things like salt, milk, and sugar, which are causing you to bloat and hold fat; and fast-burning carbs like white bread, white rice, and white potatoes, which can cause unwanted spikes in fat-storing hormones. This is what I call a *versatarian* eating program—it is versatile and emphasizes the healthiest foods, prepared simply, with the freshest flavors, herbs, and spices.

As with the fitness plan, your meal plans are color-coded, and we always start with **yellow**. On the yellow level, we'll ease into leaner, cleaner, greener eating. After that, we'll go to **orange**, where we'll get even healthier. The **blue**-level foods and recipes represent the best, cleanest, choices you can make to sustain the results you've achieved at the first two levels.

So now we're going to focus on laying the groundwork for the next 20 days. This includes some of the basic ground rules, as well as a few must-have lists that will help ensure you have all the right tools at your disposal at all times. Why is this essential? Because if you have everything you need for a healthy, 20-minute meal, you won't be running out to make last-minute, diet-sabotaging trips to the store or drive-thru.

CELEBRATION MEALS

Some diets and meal plans allow for "cheat days" or "cheat meals." I hate this idea. The second you start introducing the idea of cheating, you're sabotaging yourself. So no, you can't have a "cheat" meal. But you *can* have a "celebration meal."

Let me explain the difference. A cheat is something you haven't earned—you're cheating on your program. It sounds negative and it feels negative. But a celebration is something you've earned through hard work. That's what you get to have on my program.

Can you give me 10 days of really great nutrition and exercise? *Can I get just 10 days out of you, please?* That's not a ton of time, but it's definitely enough for you to start noticing a difference in your body. If you can give me 10 days of awesome, I'll hand you a celebration meal that you can have on the evening of Day 10, midway through your 20-day program.

- **YELLOW:** Start your meal with a vegetable salad and a healthy dressing. Order a dish you're really craving and split it with a friend. Enjoy a maximum of one of each of the following: one alcoholic beverage (5 ounces of wine, a 4-ounce cocktail, or a 12-ounce beer), one serving of bread from the bread basket (one slice of bread, or one normal-size roll, without butter), and half a dessert (share it with a friend). Enjoy your meal. Savor it. Then go home, stretch, relax, and set your alarm to get up bright and early and back to your program.

- **ORANGE:** Same as yellow, with one change: enjoy *two* out of three of the bread, alcohol, and dessert. (Did you notice that the initial letters of those three words spell BAD?)

- **BLUE:** Same as yellow, with one change: enjoy *one* out of three of the bread, alcohol, and dessert.

A celebration meal is an acknowledgment that sometimes food is fun and you can absolutely treat yourself occasionally to things that you won't base your diet on year-round. If you plan it well, a treat becomes a celebration that won't derail your efforts.

Allow yourself a celebration meal every 10 days or so. Just be sure to stay honest with yourself. Don't eat so much that you're bloated and uncomfortable; eat just until you feel satisfied. Enjoy your celebration and know that it's now an occasional part of your life to be savored, not a cheat to feel guilty about.

EMPTY CALORIES AND ALCOHOL

I live in Los Angeles and believe me, the nightlife here is awesome! But it's also risky because it's so easy to fill your nights going out with friends and doing things that might trip up your program, such as drinking too much.

Alcohol is the ultimate empty calorie. When people ask me for tips on how to lose weight, I tell them that the number one thing to cut down on is alcohol. Alcohol turns right into sugar when it hits your liver. And a "wine pour" at most restaurants is much larger than the recommended five ounces. It's like eating an extra meal at midnight and still expecting to lose weight. In other words, it's not going to happen.

Alcohol is also risky because our bodies naturally want to eat when we're drinking, in order to absorb and metabolize the alcohol. That can lead to more unwanted calories. The worst decisions typically happen when we drink. Be honest: when was the last time you showed up sober at 2 a.m. for pancakes at IHOP?

I'm not asking you to give up alcohol completely, but I am asking you to be really honest about how much you drink if you want to lose weight. Here are my tips for enjoying alcohol in a way that will minimize its impact on your body over the next 20 days.

- Decide before you go out how much you're going to drink or if you're going to drink at all. If you are drinking to be social, set a strict limit: I'd say one drink for women and two drinks for men will be more than enough if you're seriously committed to your weight loss.

- Don't drink too late into the evening or you won't sleep well because you'll be waking up in the middle of the night to go to the bathroom and because alcohol interrupts natural sleep cycles.

- Red wine is one of the better options because it contains compounds that may promote heart health. A glass of wine generally has less sugar than a standard four-ounce well drink and a four-ounce well drink is usually less sugary than sweet cocktails, which are packed with calories. A four-ounce mai tai—which is a blend of lime juice, curaçao, light and dark rum—can contain 250 or more calories and 18 grams of sugar,[28] while a five-ounce "pour" of red wine has about 125 calories and less than five grams of sugar.[29]

- Lighter-colored alcoholic drinks are "cleaner," but it's still important to gulp water between drinks so that you don't get too tipsy and accidentally overindulge. Drinking water also keeps your stomach full, which will help prevent the late-night drive-thru run that often punctuates a night out on the town. Don't use alcohol as a "vacation from stress." That's like putting a Band-Aid on a gunshot wound. Find healthy, sustainable ways to deal with stress. And one great way to burn off that stress? You guessed it: exercise.

STAYING HYDRATED

It's just as important to drink enough water (or other nonalcoholic fluids) during the day as it is to eat well. Adequate water consumption helps you to stay hydrated and it maximizes countless other bodily functions, such as brain activity and metabolism.

If you can, carry with you, throughout the day, a thermos or reusable water bottle that you can refill. The National Academy of Sports Medicine recommends that you drink half your bodyweight in ounces of water each day. For example, a 120-pound woman would drink 60 ounces of water daily from all sources, including tea, coffee, and even fruit and veggies. If water isn't your favorite beverage, try unsweetened iced tea (preferably green tea) or squeeze some lemon or other sliced fruit into your water. Having enough water also helps your body to retain less water, so you'll experience less bloating. Finally, water can help you suppress cravings by keeping you full. Studies show that consuming 16 ounces of water before a meal can help you eat fewer calories!

When it comes to other beverages, I advise staying away from diet sodas, which are full of chemicals. Diet soda can also stimulate your sweet tooth, leading you to overeat other sweet foods. And if you want a flat stomach, consider avoiding not only diet soft drinks but all carbonated beverages, which can make you bloated and gassy.

Why not replace diet soda with a more satisfying beverage? Try a mix of iced herbal tea, stevia (a natural sweetener), and seltzer to start. It's sweet and cold and fizzy and free of all the artificial flavors and sweeteners. From there, take out the seltzer and just drink stevia-sweetened iced tea. Finally, try unsweetened herbal or green iced tea all by itself or with a squeeze of lemon. You'll knock yourself off that diet soda habit in no time.

SUPPLEMENTING YOUR NUTRITION

Nutritional supplements are not required for the *20-Minute Body* program, but I highly recommend taking a few to help your body recover properly from your workouts. Here's the list of supplements that I use regularly and recommend to my clients:

Fish oil

Plant-based protein powder

Green drink powder

A probiotic to promote good digestion

Glutamine and branched chain amino acids (BCAAs)

Make sure you take them only as directed, and shop around to make sure you're getting the highest-quality product that you can afford.

THE 20-MINUTE PANTRY

While fresh, perishable items like meats and produce are the main staples that you'll use to fuel workouts and lose inches and pounds, it's also important to keep a well-stocked pantry to ensure that you always have the ingredients to make a healthy meal.

This does end up being somewhat of a tricky area for most people because when it comes to your dry groceries—your pastas, rice, and tortillas, for example—you are probably used to certain brands, certain flavors, and, yes, certain prices. But as we've discussed, a great majority of these foods are full of chemicals and preservatives that can counteract the hard work you're putting in elsewhere. That's why it's necessary to first rid your pantry of things that aren't beneficial for your health. Yes, even those breakfast cereals. Start with the ones that have a cartoon character on the box and sugar as the first ingredient and work your way out from there!

Your 20-Minute Pantry will still contain many familiar foods, just in healthier forms. When it comes to bread, for example, look for whole wheat and whole-grain versions. If the first ingredient on the label is anything besides "whole wheat flour," put it back.

And pasta isn't off-limits, either. These days, there are plenty of whole-grain options available and you can use the same label sense as when you buy your bread to get a healthier, higher-fiber alternative than traditional pasta.

Complement these mainstays with other nutrient-rich choices like brown rice, nuts, black beans, tomato paste, and low-sodium broth, and you'll have a decked-out, health-first pantry with options galore.

Here are the *20-Minute Body* Pantry Staples. You will use these ingredients in the meal plans that follow in Chapter 12:

1 small bag whole wheat or whole-grain bread crumbs

2 small whole wheat or whole-grain pitas

4 whole wheat 100-calorie sandwich flats

12 corn taco shells, small corn tortillas, or whole-grain soft tortillas

Eight 6-inch whole wheat or whole-grain flour tortillas

1 loaf whole wheat or whole-grain bread

One 42-ounce container old-fashioned oats

One 16-oounce bag shredded unsweetened flaked coconut

One 8-ounce box whole wheat or whole-grain pasta

One 8-ounce box whole wheat or whole-grain spaghetti

One 14-ounce box instant brown rice

One 16-ounce bag chia seeds

One 16-ounce bag ground flaxseed

One 12-ounce box raisins

One pound box brown sugar

80-count bag of Stevia or 1 bag of Stevia granules

One 8-ounce bag walnuts

CANNED JARRED GOODS

One 15-ounce can pumpkin

One 5-ounce can chipotle peppers in adobe sauce

Two 5-ounce cans tomato paste

Two 15-ounce cans diced tomatoes

Two 15-ounce cans low-sodium beans

One 15-ounce can chickpeas

One 15-ounce can black beans

One 10-ounce container pitted olives

Two 32-ounce containers low-sodium chicken or vegetable broth

TOP 20 HERBS AND SPICES

People love to use salty or sweet flavors to spruce up otherwise healthy food. That tangy barbeque sauce you use on your chicken breasts or that aggressive work with the salt shaker to spruce up your veggies . . . these are pretty commonplace practices, even for people who think they're eating healthy. You can do better for yourself *without* compromising on taste. There are so many flavors out there to explore that do more than liven up bland dishes—they're actually better for you, either because they omit harmful white stuff, or include other health-rich compounds, or both. Fresh or dried herbs and spices not only add tons of flavor to your foods (without adding salt or oil) but also have a host of health benefits of their own. So take a look at your spice cabinet, note what you already have on our top 20 list, and then stock up the remaining herbs and spices on the list—you will be using them all in the 20-minute recipes!

SPICES

BLACK PEPPERCORNS add peppery taste to any meal. Freshly grinding your pepper in a pepper mill or coffee grinder is the best way to bring out its flavor (pre-ground pepper tends to lose its spark sitting on the grocery store shelf).

CARDAMOM, a spice that resembles black pepper, has a minty flavor. Take your knowledge of seasoning to the next level with ground cardamom by using a pinch in desserts and sweet breakfast foods for a hint of the exotic.

CHILI POWDER is an easy way to get out of a bland cooking rut. Look for chili powder that is mild to hot, salt-free, and sugar-free. Start with mild chili powder and gradually add pinches of hotter ground chili, such as cayenne, to build your tolerance to the heat.

CHIPOTLE CHILE PEPPERS in adobo sauce heat up your metabolism and tingle your taste buds, and they also happen to be rich in antioxidants and vitamins, including vitamin C.

CHILI FLAKES, made up of chopped dried chilies and seeds, are a grocery store standard. They're perfect to perk up Italian fare. Add them to jarred marinara sauce for a zesty flavor boost. Capsaicin, the compound found in chili peppers that gives them their heat, can also aid in fat-burning while lowering blood pressure.

CINNAMON, a much-loved American spice, is ideal for breakfast foods like hot cereals, French toast, and smoothies. Sweet-tasting cinnamon may actually help control blood sugar spikes, so it is an ideal companion at breakfast time, when leveled blood sugar can help to break your morning haze more quickly. Cinnamon has also been correlated with lower levels of inflammation.

CITRUS ZEST isn't officially an herb or a spice, but it adds such bright flavor to meat mixtures, fish, and spice mixes that I can't resist recommending it here. Some studies say that citrus zest may be protective against certain forms of cancer, like skin cancer.

CUMIN gives Latin fare its characteristic tang. It is surprisingly high in iron compared with other spices. Be cautious with the amount since the flavor can be overpowering. Try using cumin seeds that you can grind yourself, or toast in a warm dry skillet for a gourmet garnish.

FENNEL SEEDS, often used in ground sausage, give off a sweet licorice taste that doesn't require any added sugar. Grind fennel seeds in spice mixes to contrast with spicy chilies or add them toasted to bean mixtures or taco meat.

GARLIC POWDER is a fast and flavorful way to get that garlicky taste—no mincing required! Be sure to pick up garlic powder and not garlic salt, which adds unwanted sodium.

GROUND GINGER, milder in flavor than fresh gingerroot, is typically used in gingerbread cookies and curry mixes. It works equally well in savory dishes and is a base component in Chef Rocco's spice mix or in a tangy homemade salad dressing.

HERBS

BASIL paired with fresh tomatoes or as a sprig added to your favorite marinara sauce is just about the best thing going. Basil has fresh flavor and a few interesting health benefits—it may calm blood pressure and relax the nervous system.

CHIVES, part of the onion genus, have a mild flavor that is perfect with eggs, in dips, or sprinkled over white fish or shellfish.

CILANTRO, a lemony floral-flavored herb, is popular in cooking around the globe including Mexican, Thai, and Indian cuisines. Cilantro, like rosemary, has antibacterial properties that may ward off food poisoning.

CORIANDER is the seed of the cilantro plant. Grind the seeds with cumin or chili powder for a savory mix for ground meat, or add powdered coriander to hot chocolate for a great flavor boost.

MINT is delicious in smoothies combined with greens like spinach and kale. If you have leftover mint, simply pour hot water over the fresh leaves for a refreshing calorie-free tea.

PARSLEY, rich in vitamin K (important for bone health), is a fresh herb that's easy to find year-round. Flat-leaf parsley has more flavor and is easier to chop than other varieties.

THYME's earthy flavor perks up almost any dish: stews, bean mixtures, mashes, and soups. Thyme has a strong taste, so use smaller amounts (about 1 teaspoon fresh thyme leaves to start).

ROSEMARY, part of the mint family, is savory added to seasoning salts, in meat marinades, and combined with vinegars like balsamic or sherry. Like thyme, rosemary contains antibacterial compounds and is used in the meat industry as a natural, safe preservative. It has also been correlated with better heart health and lowered cancer risk.

OREGANO is packed with antioxidants, which help prevent cell damage. Dried oregano is found in herb mixtures like Italian seasonings and herbs de Provence. Add a pinch when cooking onions and vegetables or sprinkle some into the calzone recipe on page 254 or the pizza recipe on page 301.

20-MINUTE KITCHEN TOOLS

Watching my friend Chef Rocco do his thing in his kitchen, I am amazed at the many tools he uses to create his culinary masterpieces. But each one has its purpose. We can't all be Chef Rocco, but the good news is we don't need to be. By adding some key tools to your own kitchen, you can do everything you need to prepare meals that are ingredient-minimal but packed with flavor. This list includes the basics, and some of them are probably already in your kitchen.

INEXPENSIVE ESSENTIALS

A SET OF TONGS that are light and easy to handle will make cooking proteins and veggies a snap. They're also dishwasher safe for easy cleanup.

A SET OF THREE PLASTIC CUTTING BOARDS: These boards are inexpensive and wash in the dishwasher easily.

A VEGETABLE PEELER. The Swissmar Peeler, light and ultrasharp, will peel through tough potato skins and delicate fruit peels. To protect the blades, hand-wash with soap and water.

A DISHWASHER-SAFE SLICER for homemade sweet potato chips and squash noodles.

A SPATULA. The ideal spatula has a slender and flexible edge to easily slide underneath fish, eggs, or your other skillet creations.

A MICROPLANE. Use it to grate nutmeg, garlic cloves, and citrus zest. Slide it into your dishwasher for easy cleanup.

KITCHEN SHEARS can snip herbs or even cut a chicken breast into tenders in a snap. Stainless-steel blades make them dishwasher safe and the blades come apart for easier clean-up.

TWO SKILLETS (LARGE AND SMALL) are all you'll need to make many of the recipes in this book. The tough stainless-steel skillets made by All-Clad will last a lifetime.

A CAST-IRON SKILLET that's easy to handle and clean.

 A COFFEE GRINDER does more than just grind coffee beans: it's also ideal for grinding fresh spices, as well as for making your own oat flour from old-fashioned oats.

 3 BASIC KNIVES: an 8-inch chef's knife, a serrated knife, and a paring knife.

 TUPPERWARE for storing your food in a way that makes refrigerator organizing easier and allows you to grab food and go.

 MEASURING CUPS AND SPOONS that allow you to get super-precise with your food prep and flavoring.

 A THERMOS that can keep smoothies cold.

 A REUSABLE WATER BOTTLE that can help you make sure you're drinking enough water during the day.

DREAM HEALTHY KITCHEN ITEMS

The listed kitchen appliances below make healthy cooking quick and easy, though some are more of an investment than others. Keep an eye out for sales, or ask for one of these on your Christmas or birthday wish list!

 AN IMMERSION BLENDER blends soups right in the stockpot. This model also comes with attachments that allows it to double as a mini-chopper and an electric whisk. It's also great for blending sauces and salad dressings.

 A FOOD PROCESSOR will cut your prep time in half for everything from mixing pizza dough to chopping, dicing, and shredding your favorite veggies.

 THE NINJA PROFESSIONAL BLENDER has a powerful motor that won't stop until your smoothies, veggies, and ice-based creations are silky smooth.

 A SLOW COOKER cooks for you! Prep for less than 20 minutes in the morning, turn it on, and by the time you're home for dinner you'll have a warm meal.

 NUTRIGRILL (OR OTHER PORTABLE GRILL-TOP APPLIANCE) for grilling anything healthfully and quickly with less cleanup.

 OPTIONAL: A digital food scale for ultra-accurate portion measurements is very handy to have until you can start to eyeball portions from experience.

CLEANER, LEANER, AND GREENER

Put these additional eating strategies to work to drop inches even faster!

TAPER OFF. Dinner should be the last time you eat in the evening. You need less fuel at the end of the day because you're less active, so any extra calories you take in are more likely to be stored as fat.

SNACK WISE. Had a teeny-tiny dinner? You can nosh in the late evening but keep it small—like a bowl of oatmeal or veggies and hummus.

STOCK UP AT WORK. Wherever you spend most of your time is where most of your food needs to be. If you're at work all day, you can avoid trips to the vending machine or lunch truck by stocking your drawer or office fridge with healthy snacks.

FIGHT CRAVINGS. Having a snack between meals, especially a high-fiber snack, helps stabilize your blood sugar and prevent crashes.

GO H_2O: Try to drink half of your bodyweight in ounces of water per day. For example, if you weigh 150 pounds, drink 75 ounces of water per day. Carry a thermos or reusable water bottle with you so you know how much to drink. Drinking an adequate amount of water will help to nullify cravings.

DON'T SKIP MEALS. Skipping meals, which is advocated on some diet plans, causes a drop in your blood sugar, which usually leads to excessive hunger and then overeating. You can also slow down and even damage your metabolism by repeatedly putting your body into a "famine" state by not eating.

DON'T SKIP BREAKFAST . . . EVER. Many people skip breakfast and then eat two large meals a day. The combination of eating large portions but eating less often boosts insulin production, which increases fat storage.

PREPPED FOR SUCCESS

You've committed to losing a few pounds, and what better time to start your new workout plan and nutritional discipline than a Monday, right? So you head to work and—surprise!—Monday just owns you. Before you know it, the workload has piled up and now you're not even going to make it out of the office on time. One gruesome commute later, you finally drag yourself back into the house. It's late, you're beat, and the last thing you want to do is stand over the stove to prepare your planned meal of chicken, sweet potato, and asparagus. Time to rummage through the pans, pull out the chicken, get the oven warm. At this point, you decide that the best time to start your diet is—as ever—tomorrow.

You see, while you can't always plan out how your workday is going to go or what each day will throw at you, you can invest a little bit more time to make sure that you have all the essentials in place and that you're in a position each and every day to succeed in the kitchen.

Meal preparation is one of the most daunting things for people when it comes to living a healthier lifestyle. Cooking high-flavor, body-friendly foods takes time, but if you put into practice the tips that I've laid out in this chapter, it will take far less. Don't fall into the Monday trap—do your prep work the night before and make sure you have all of your groceries on hand so that you can hit the ground running on Monday night. When you start getting into the mindset that healthy living doesn't have to be a hassle, you'll find that losing weight is a lot easier and much less of a chore.

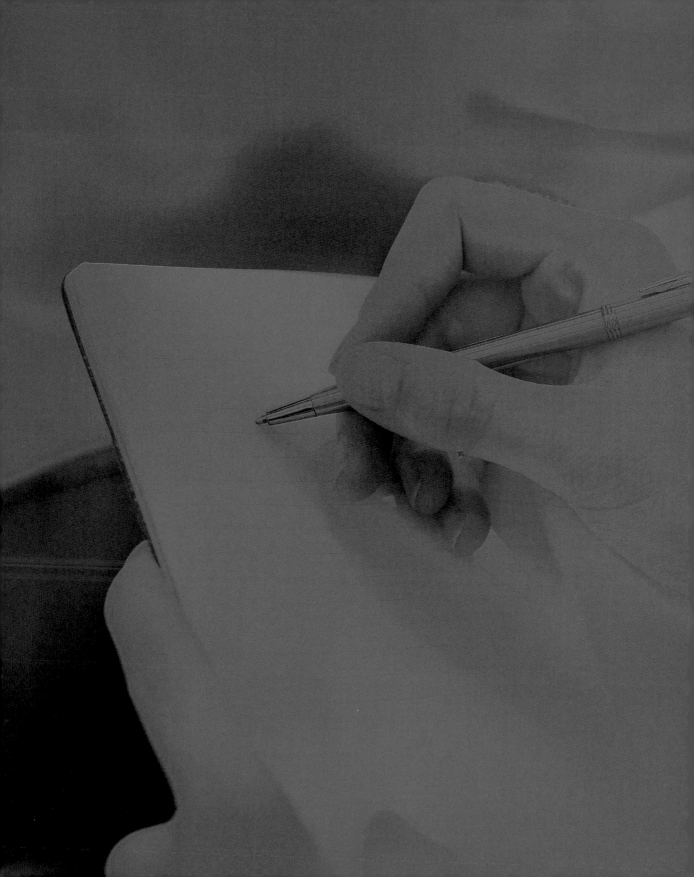

TEN

The 20-Day Mindset Plan

O NE OF THE MOST DISTINGUISHING aspects of the *20-Minute Body* pro-gram is that you'll be spending 20 minutes each week training your brain to sustain you in your journey to a leaner body. The color levels are not as relevant to this portion of your training. But if you expect to continue building on good habits and reinforcing your "why," it's import-ant to constantly train in this area, always pushing yourself to do more, to be better. For example, once you have a firmer understanding of the challenges that you need to overcome, you may decide to reassess your goal-setting in Week 2 or Week 3. But you won't know to do that if you aren't journaling regularly and doing your mind training. I want you to spend a few minutes a day, working toward 20 minutes per week, focusing on these activities. Do not skip this part of the program! Your success rests on your adherence to daily mindset training.

Learning how to strengthen yourself from within is a very personal journey, but setting aside a few minutes each day to devote to that jour-ney is essential. Some folks may write down a goal at the beginning of a weight loss program—"I want to lose 20 pounds," for example—but then they bury it, or it simply becomes lost in all of the new sets, reps, meals, and snacks they are focused on. And then, real life creeps into your fitness life. Your kids require your attention, work is pulling you in a thousand different directions, you have your anniversary to plan, that family vacation has been on the books for months, you have a falling-out with a friend, an unexpected bill comes in the mail, a neighbor needs your help . . . and the list goes on. All of these things can create stress and distract you from your goals. And if you don't have the proper mindset, their collective weight starts to feel overwhelming. Suddenly, those clean meals you've been wanting to prepare are less important. Your regular workout times are intruded upon. *Fitness can wait another day*, you say to yourself. You start falling back on old excuses. False mantras like "The best day to start a new fitness routine is always tomorrow" start to take root in your psyche, condemning you to yet another failed attempt at getting those inches off.

This doesn't happen if you have *fitness from within*. And that is cultivated by spending just a few minutes each day focusing your mind, bringing your objectives and motivations into focus, identifying and snuffing out weaknesses or deficiencies in your planning, or even just thinking about the work that lies ahead of you. If you dedicate yourself to this practice each day, I guarantee that you will be far more likely to change your body for life and change the life of your body.

SMART GOALS AND JOURNALING

The first thing to do when starting out is to ask yourself a fundamental question: *Do I know my goals and what I really want to accomplish physically, mentally, and emotionally?* You might just want to dive right into the meal plans and workouts, but without proper attention to goal setting, you'll be ill-equipped to measure your progress or stay motivated along the way. Setting goals is something that is very important to me; and for every client I train, this is where we start. You might be thinking, "Well, I picked up your book, so clearly my goal is to lose weight." That's fair, but I want you to have a deeper understanding and appreciation of the process, not just the payoff.

I want you to consider what it really takes to set a goal. *SMART* is a good acronym to remember when it comes to goal-setting, because it describes all the elements of a well-set goal.

S—Specific
M—Measurable
A—Achievable
R—Realistic
T—Timely

By constantly setting goals for yourself that meet these criteria, you are able to build a habit of success, which builds confidence, which keeps you working harder and harder. Before you know it, you'll be setting goals for yourself that are bigger than anything you could have thought possible.

Try to set goals for yourself that are "action goals." An action goal is one that you achieve through action, like "My goal is to complete all of my *20-Minute Body* workouts by 8 a.m. each day this week." That's a goal that is completely under your control. If you choose a results-based goal like "I will lose 20 inches in 20 days no matter what," you're setting yourself up for disappointment if for some reason your body doesn't go along with your wishes. If you want to lose 20 inches, this program will get you there. But it may take longer than you want it to, so focusing on what you can control will keep you motivated and moving in the right direction. In the mindset exercises, we'll revisit goal-setting frequently—reevaluating and adjusting goals is not a bad thing—but it's important to establish right now exactly *how* those goals should be formed so that you give yourself the best chance to notch "small" successes along the way to your 20 inches, or whatever goal you are working toward.

THE IMPORTANCE OF JOURNALING

To know where you're going, it's a good idea to know where you are and where you've been. That's why keeping a journal is such an important part of any weight loss program. This may sound like homework, or something else to learn, but remember that I want this to be an easy, enjoyable process. So rest assured that while I will be giving you suggestions, I won't be locking you into any kind of rigid journaling format.

A journal is a way for you to track your daily progress in the three main areas: fitness, nutrition, and mindset. What you keep track of is entirely up to you, but here are some things you can monitor through a good journal:

FITNESS

Reps done

Weight used

How you felt post-workout

How a particular exercise felt

How much of your allotted rest you actually used

Your rate of perceived exertion (see Chapter 6)

How much you liked a workout

Challenges you faced with certain exercises or sets

Moves where you felt you could have pushed harder

Your soreness level

NUTRITION

Favorite foods

Foods you can get "cleaner" on

Food temptations at work, school, home

The times of your meals

The amount of each food on your plate (protein, starch, greens)

How a particular meal made you feel (satisfied, bloated, etc.)

How a certain recipe tasted

Recipes you want to try tomorrow

Your energy levels after certain meals or foods

Things you can do better with prep

MINDSET

Your SMART goals

What time you're setting aside for mindset training

Whether you felt this time was productive

Your confidence level

Your ability to focus

Your actual mindset exercises

Ideas on building accountability

Identifying new sources of inspiration and motivation

Coming up with new mantras

Your feelings about how you are progressing overall

When you record your progress regularly, you can use it as a reference to guide the days ahead. You might find that you did 12 reps of a particular exercise, but you noted that you thought you could do more. Great. Today, put that note to the test and go for it. The journal is a crystal ball of sorts. You might correlate one of your meals with a subpar workout, or connect a bad night's sleep to a slip-up on your eating plan. The presence of a journal helps you stay accountable to yourself.

Share your successes and struggles, or any part of your journal, with the rest of the *20-Minute Body* community on Facebook at https://www.facebook.com/20MinuteBody.

I like to use an old-fashioned paper notebook for a journal, though some people may choose to keep a journal on their smartphone, in a blog, or through some other digital format, and that's okay, too. Whatever tracking system you choose, keep it simple enough that you'll have time to use it consistently. Track the things that matter most to you. Just make sure you're keeping as much information as possible so that when you go back to reference something, you can learn from your mistakes, marvel at your successes, and feel confident about how much knowledge of yourself and your body you have gained.

THE JOURNEY TOWARD FITNESS FROM WITHIN

As with any new process, you have to start somewhere. In the beginning, your mindset training will feel very mechanical. That's okay. You have to learn what it's like to write down goals, how to keep a journal, what your best internal motivators are. But before long, these things will start to feel more natural, more intuitive. No longer just "exercises," your mindset time will start to feel more like an extension of yourself—just another instinctive task, like brushing your teeth or getting dressed for work.

We're going to start with some exercises that allow you to assess and identify your motivations and goals, while also creating a framework of accountability. These things are so important when you are starting out a new fitness journey because they allow you to get in touch with yourself and create a support structure. While *fitness from within* is your ultimate goal, having others around you to encourage and inspire you when things get hard is an incredibly valuable gift.

After these base-building exercises have been done you can start to really grow your mental muscle by reinforcing your "why," reassessing goals, and rewarding yourself for your efforts. Consistently applying these practices helps you to forge the mental muscle that you will carry with you for life.

If you follow the fitness and nutrition plans beyond the first 20 days, you'll get even more opportunities to bolster your brain. After a couple of 20-day programs, you're going to be very dialed in to how you've kept yourself motivated throughout the ups and downs of this program. You probably will have noticed some great insights during your mindset training that will help you to keep focused and dedicated for the long haul.

As you move through these exercises, keep in mind your long-term goals. What shifts in your mindset, your habits, or your daily schedule will be necessary to make your healthy lifestyle a *long-term habit*? If you look back years from now, what decisions will you have made in this initial 20-day period that will have led you to a healthier you?

GETTING STARTED

You'll perform these mindset exercises each day at a time of your choosing, for the length of time that you have available. This can come before your workouts, on your lunch break, or even just before bed—whatever is most suitable for your lifestyle and schedule. The important thing is to secure a space that is quiet—a place where you can achieve the kind of focus that's needed to cement your mantras and solidify your resolve. It may help to don a set of headphones and listen to music that calms you down—whatever helps you narrow your focus for the few minutes that I'm asking you to set aside for these crucial exercises.

Use this day-by-day guide throughout your first 20 days. As I said, it might feel a bit mechanical at first, but it is important to experiment with these exercises so that you can freestyle a bit—choosing what works for you and modifying or even discarding what doesn't work—as you continue on your journey.

DAY 1: TAKE STOCK

Take a few minutes to write out your thoughts about where you are now in your life. How do you feel during the day? Do you have a lot of energy, or are you tired all the time? How are you sleeping at night? What specific changes would you like to see in your body, energy level, and mindset over the next 20 days?

Think about what you accomplished today. I hope you had a kick-butt workout and a delicious, healthy meal. How did these things make you feel?

Take a moment to write down your personal commitment to finishing —to seeing all 20 days through to the end. Commit to doing whatever it takes to complete the 20 days.

DAY 2: FINDING YOUR "WHY"

Take a few minutes to review your workout and meals for the day. Set an intention for yourself for this day. What's the one thing you most want to accomplish? Or if the day is over, focus on tomorrow's goals.

Before your program began, I asked you to think about this question: What's your "why?" Why are you committing yourself to this program now? Take the time to identify your deepest motivations and write down your thoughts.

Now, choose a photo that describes your "why" and that you can post in a place where you'll see it—your bathroom mirror, the fridge, on top of your coffeemaker. It can be anything. A family member? A photo of your mantra? A place you want to visit when you're fit and healthy? Make it visible. Make sure you can really *feel* it!

Take a last moment before hitting the sack today to think about this: I know you're sore. I'm sure of it. These workouts aren't supposed to be easy. And you know what? You're probably going to be sore tomorrow, too. That's part of the process of waking your body up and challenging yourself. Acknowledge the soreness, the tiredness, and whatever else you're feeling. Those are your muscles and they did amazing things for you today! And you can make them do amazing things tomorrow.

DAY 3: GET SMART

Consider what it really takes to set a goal. SMART goals are the ones that are *specific, measurable, achievable, realistic,* and *timely.* Write down one SMART goal for yourself now that you've had a couple of days to get used to working out daily and preparing healthy meals.

DAY 4: START A PHOTO FOOD JOURNAL

Keeping a food journal is a great way to track what you're eating and when you're trying new foods (and how you like them). It's also great for making notes about new recipes and flavors to try. Today, I'd like you to consider trying a photo journal for tracking your meals. Take a photo of one or more of your healthy meals and post it to your social media sites, with a hashtag, to inspire your friends to try it, too.

What meals have you really enjoyed so far?

DAY 5: GO SOCIAL!

Yesterday I asked you to post a photo of a healthy meal with a hashtag to your social media sites. Today, let's take that a step further. By sharing your goals with your friends, you'll inspire them to get started on a great health goal of their own. Today, create a hashtag for yourself that captures your own personal health journey. (Here are a few of my favorites: #FitnessFromWithin, #SharingIsCaring, #AspireToInspire.) Use that hashtag from now until the end of your 20-day program whenever you're posting news about your program on your social media sites.

What hashtag have you chosen and why?

DAY 6: FOCUS ON SLEEP

Have you noticed a difference in the way you are sleeping since beginning the *20-Minute Body* program? Sleep is a huge part of our health. It affects every system in our bodies, including the systems that regulate how hungry we are.[30]

Take a moment to consider how you are sleeping. Are you getting enough sleep nightly? Are there things you could do to create a more peaceful sleeping environment for yourself? Write down your thoughts and identify one thing you can do to help yourself have more restful sleep (like putting your tablet or other electronic devices in a room other than your bedroom, stretching before bed, or having a cup of herbal tea and unwinding a half hour before your usual bedtime).

DAY 7: REST ACTIVELY

Congratulations! You've made it to the end of your first week. Today is a required rest day, but instead of sitting on the couch, why not rest actively? Today, I'd like you to try a completely new activity—nothing strenuous, but something that's just a bit "out of the box" for you. This could be anything from a pick up softball game with your kids to going to a restorative yoga class to taking a walk in the park with your spouse. Today is your day to relax and enjoy an activity for the fun of it. Whatever you choose to do, make it something that feels fresh, new, and interesting to you.

DAY 8: PICTURE THIS, AND A NEW MANTRA

This is the beginning of Week 2. For many people, this is when their enthusiasm and commitment begin to wane and the negative voices start to pipe up. Fight through that chatter by choosing a new mantra for the week. You made it through last week—let's take this week by storm!

You've probably guessed that I'm a big fan of social media. Today, take a photo of yourself after a workout and post it to your social media with an inspiring message. Tag a friend who you think would be inspired to work out because of your "nudge."

DAY 9: GRATITUDE

What are you grateful for today? Take time today to write down five things you're truly grateful for. Add a sentence or two describing why each of your five choices is important to you.

DAY 10: A NEW FITNESS TEST, AND CELEBRATIONS!

Take your fitness assessment again. Write down your results. Do you see any improvements in your overall fitness level?

If you'd like to have a planned "celebration" meal today, go for it. Be sure to write down what celebration you chose, and how you did it in a way that would help you get right back to your program *immediately* afterward.

DAY 11: AN "OUT OF THE BOX" GOAL

Start to think about an "out of the box" goal. That's something outside your health and fitness goals that you want to accomplish (not necessarily in 20 days). In fact, it might be something you've always dreamed of doing but never thought you could accomplish, until now. Fitness and health are great things to strive for because you get stronger and more confident in every area of your life.

DAY 12: NEW TASTES

Are you discovering new favorite foods as a result of the *20-Minute Body* eating program? Write down the ones you've tried so far that you really like. Have any of them surprised you? Keep track of your new favorite tastes, your favorite new recipes, and things you'd like to try more of in the future.

DAY 13: TIME MANAGEMENT

How are you spending your time? I bet that before this program started, you wondered how you could really increase your fitness and lose weight just by exercising for 20 minutes a day and making meals in 20 minutes or less. But I also think that by now, you've realized that you can get a lot of things done in 20 minutes, as long as you're *completely focused* on your goal.

Today, take stock of how you spend your time, especially if you'd like to tackle a larger goal that takes more time than you think you have. Pay special attention to your "screen time" —that's the time you spend in front of a smartphone, tablet, or computer that isn't related to work. One great way to find more time in your day is to reduce the amount of downtime you spend doing sedentary things like watching TV or going online.

Write down how much aimless time today you spent in front of screens, and try to reduce that time by 10 percent this week.

DAY 14: YOUR SECOND "ACTIVE REST"

Congratulations! You've reached the end of your second week and have arrived at your second required rest day. Maybe you want to go back to the same activity you tried last week . . . or maybe you'd like to try something new. The important thing is to move and enjoy yourself.

Write down what you did and how you felt.

DAY 15: NEW FLAVORS, NEW MANTRAS

It's the beginning of Week 3. This is the time when some people might start to backslide on nutrition. Be prepared to head that off at the pass by trying new flavors, spices, and tastes. Try a new recipe or, using what you've learned so far, improvise your own! Decide on a new mantra for this week as well, and a new hashtag to go with it.

DAY 16: NUTRITION "PROGRESSIONS"

Look at the ideas for nutrition progressions in Chapter 12. What progressions have you come up with for your program to improve your nutrition over time? Map out your own nutrition progression on paper. Draw out exactly what you've done to get from where you were to where you are now.

DAY 17: PUSHING THROUGH SETBACKS

By now, you've been working hard for two full weeks. It's easy to have a few good days of health but consistency is the hard part. Maybe you've had a meal that was "off plan" or missed a workout or just went through a day feeling sluggish. It happens to everyone. But you're still here, and that's a big accomplishment. Every time you practice what you're going to do when things get hard, you actually figure out how to keep going when things get hard. Mental reps. Make sense? You do it just by doing it. Write down a setback or challenge you've experienced thus far, and what you did to overcome it.

DAY 18: CHANGING CRAVINGS

How have your cravings changed since you began this program? Are you noticing new cravings for healthier foods? Has your desire for salty or sugary foods subsided? As you improve the quality of your nutrition, you will naturally start to crave wholesome foods because your body will be looking for those nutrients.

Take time today to note the types of cravings you've been having and whether they have changed since the beginning of your program. If you've still been craving bad stuff, note that as well. Evaluate whether those cravings hit you while you were engaged in one of your food triggers, like staying up late, watching TV, or sitting in front of the computer.

DAY 19: YOUR "HEALTHY HIT LIST"

Over the past 19 days, you've had a chance to really notice improvements in all areas of your health. Now, here's a chance for you to create a "healthy hit list"—a list of the changes that have been the most noticeable and meaningful to you.

Your "healthy hit list" will be personal to you—no two people's lists will look alike. What positive change have you noticed? It could be the way your clothes fit, the amount of energy you have, the quality of your sleep, or the spring in your step during that time in the afternoon when you used to get tired. Or it could be an overall sense of happiness, a renewed focus, a sense of optimism about your life, or a decrease in unhealthy habits like getting irritable or snacking on the wrong things late at night.

Update this list going forward as you continue to notice positive changes.

DAY 20: CELEBRATE!

It's time to celebrate! You've reached the end of your first 20 days. Take a few moments to express your gratitude and describe your celebration, in writing. What are you thankful for today? How has this program helped you to become more aware of the things you're grateful for in your life?

If you'd like, plan a celebration meal (again, using the guidelines in Chapter 9). And reward yourself in other, non-food ways. How about a massage for your sore muscles, or a new piece of workout clothing, or a fancy boutique fitness class with a friend? Write down how you've chosen to celebrate your accomplishments.

THE MAKING OF A MINDSET

Mindset training shouldn't end when you're done with your 20-day programs. Just like muscle, your mindset can atrophy—or waste away—when you stop training. You start to forget the lessons you learned and the strength you built. You open yourself up to moments of weakness—the kind that can put you back at square one. I hope that the pages of this chapter are frayed and worn from frequent referencing. Neglecting mindset training is neglecting your commitment to yourself.

> Neglecting mindset training is neglecting your commitment to yourself.

This mindset program gives you simple and easy-to-follow exercises, each with a specific purpose. Taken together, the mindset training tips in this chapter help you inch closer *each day* to your ultimate goal.

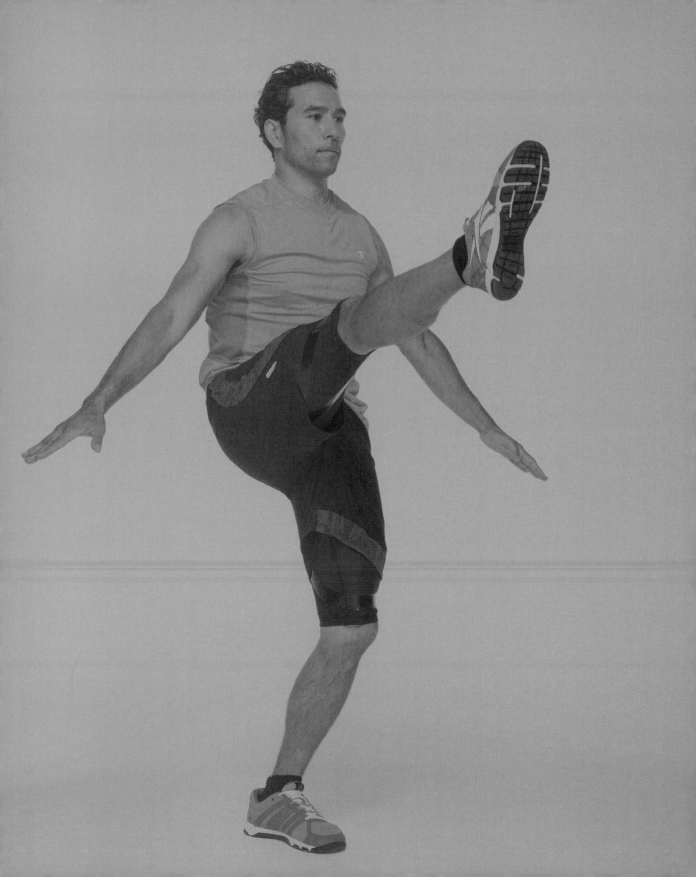

ELEVEN

The 20-Day Fitness Plan

IT'S TIME TO START TRAINING for metabolic muscle! Today will be the first day of a new way of training for you—one that gets you off that recumbent bike or treadmill and helps you find out what your body is really capable of. The goal of these workouts is simple: to help train your body to burn more fat. During your workouts, of course, you're going to burn calories—lots of 'em! —but the real prize is that your body is going to continue using energy from your fat stores long after your workouts are over.

I know you've probably put yourself through torturously long workouts at the gym before without seeing results. That's why I can't wait for you to try these workouts. It won't take long for you to see how much better off you are when you cut down your workout time to 20 minutes. By giving a max effort to every second, you will create a huge stimulus for change in your body—the harder you work, the harder it has to work during recovery. And that means more fat loss and muscle preservation along the way. And since muscle burns more calories than fat, the more you shift that ratio of fat to muscle, the more you end up converting your body into a metabolic machine, which actually becomes resistant to storing fat!

Working with me to train for metabolic muscle will be tough, but nothing is more fun or more rewarding than seeing your body do what you want it to do in less time than ever. When you start seeing the inches fall off—and believe me, they will! —you will never go back to long, slow workouts again.

THE JOURNEY

This chapter gives you the first 20 days of your new fitness approach (the yellow program) as well as the next two (orange and blue) 20-day programs to follow it up.

The best long-term workout solutions are those that account for progression: for ways to keep that challenge coming long after the introductory period. And that's what this yellow program does. Everyone will see rapid results over the course of these 20 days, and if you're new to exercise or coming back from a long layoff, those results are likely to be even more noticeable. The yellow program lays the foundation for everything that is to come and helps prepare you for orange and blue, where all of the workout variables start to get more advanced.

And because no two bodies are created equal, for each exercise listed at every stage, I'll give you options on how to make it easier or more challenging. This will allow everyone, regardless of age, skill level, or previous injury, to follow the same program. Making modifications for people is something I have to do all the time as a trainer. It's nothing to boast about if you're doing a harder version and nothing to be ashamed of if you're doing the easier one. Oftentimes, I find that the people who pick the most advanced version right off the bat have to scale back while people who do a simpler variation find that they are capable of more challenging versions. It's not about where you start—it's about where you finish.

FITNESS 101

In order to do the workouts that follow, you'll first have to learn a little fitness lingo. Don't worry; there won't be a pop quiz at the end of the chapter—and you can always turn to these pages for reference. But I actually think it's helpful for you to learn the proper terminology—after all, you are on your way to becoming a fitness pro!

FITNESS TERMS

REP: This is short for "repetition." This indicates the number of times you will perform a single exercise.

SET: A number of repetitions of a single exercise that you will do before resting, or before moving on to a set of a different exercise. Example: "Perform one set of 10 reps" means just that—perform 10 repetitions of an exercise without stopping.

SUPERSET: A group of two exercises performed back-to-back without any rest in between.

TRISET: A group of three exercises performed back-to-back-to-back without any rest in between.

When it comes to body position, movements, and grips (if you're holding an exercise band or a dumbbell), there are just a few basic terms to become familiar with.

90/90: I usually use this term to describe how to get into a proper lunging position where both knees are bent at 90-degree angles.

GRIPS: There are several ways to hold dumbbells. Here's a list of the basic grips used:

- **NEUTRAL GRIP:** Palms facing each other.
- **SUPINATED GRIP:** Palms facing up toward you. This is also called a reverse grip.

- **PRONATED GRIP:** Palms facing down.

MOVEMENTS: There are three ways to move your arms/hands or legs in an exercise. Below I've listed all three. Look for these terms in the workout descriptions.

- **BILATERAL:** Both arms or legs move together.

- **UNILATERAL:** Move only one side at a time, performing all reps on that side before switching to the other side.

- **RECIPROCAL:** Alternating sides with each rep.

ANGLE SPEAK: In addition to the positions I've listed above, you'll notice that many of the exercise names here include a letter of the alphabet: T, V, W, or Y. Those letters denote the arm position you'll use for an exercise.

THE 7 PRIMAL PATTERNS

All human movement is derived from seven primal patterns. In other words, there are only seven basic ways you can move your body. Every exercise is made up of one or more of these primal movements, which makes it easier to learn, master, and progress to more advanced exercises. One big perk of these movements is that they require the most amount of muscle.

Here's a basic guide to all seven primal movements.

1. SQUAT

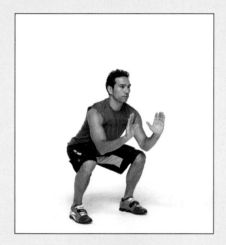

3. PUSH

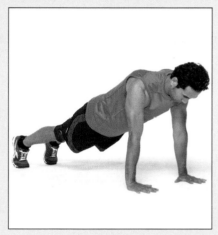

2. LUNGE

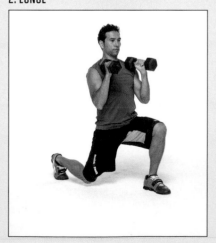

4. PULL

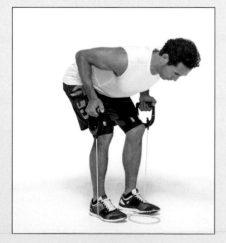

5. TWIST

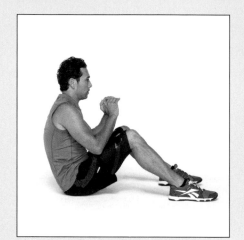

7. GAIT

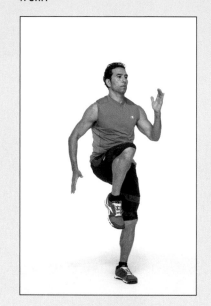

6. BEND

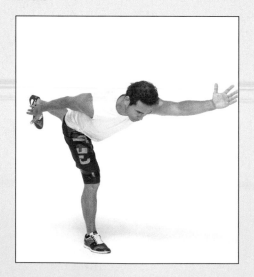

20-DAY FITNESS PLAN: YELLOW

For the next 20 days, you'll train for 20 minutes or less, working through challenging but fun routines that will produce greater results than your hour-long workouts of yesteryear. Everyone starts at yellow to ensure the best progression. Here, we'll train with five mandatory workouts, one optional workout or rest day, and one dedicated rest day each week.

Before each workout, you'll perform a short, active warm-up (see pages 90–91) to get the blood flowing and to prep your muscles for what lies ahead.

SETTING UP YOUR WORKOUT SPACE

So you've done your baseline fitness assessment and you're ready to start Day 1 of the *20-Minute Body* exercise plan. I'm sure you already have your workout clothes and your playlist, but have you even considered where you'll be doing your training?

Take a few minutes today to set up a space where you'll be able to work out each day. You need only a few feet of clear floor space and maybe an exercise mat for comfort.

It's helpful to have a full-length mirror in the room if possible. It will help you to see your posture and body position more clearly. Good posture and body position will enable you to make a strong mind-muscle connection on every rep, allowing you to get the most out of every exercise.

The most important thing? A towel. Because I'm going to make you sweat like you didn't know you could!

THE 20-DAY CALENDAR: YELLOW

Each day of the 20-day program will have you working your body in a slightly different way. This not only attacks metabolic muscle from multiple angles but also makes it nearly impossible to get bored. And if you do start to lose interest, you are always free to mix it up by trying more advanced versions of the exercises provided!

DAY	WORKOUT/ACTIVITY
1	Double Trouble
2	4x4
3	30 HI–30 LO
4	Rest, Body-Part Specific, or Cardio-Air
5	Double Trouble
6	4x4
7	Rest
8	Double Trouble
9	4x4
10	30 HI–30 LO
11	Rest, Body-Part Specific, or Cardio-Air
12	Double Trouble
13	30 HI–30 LO
14	Rest
15	Double Trouble
16	4x4
17	30 HI–30 LO
18	Rest, Body-Part Specific, or Cardio-Air
19	4x4
20	30 HI–30 LO

On days 4, 11, and 18, you have the option to perform a body-part specific (BPS) or cardio-air workout.

THE 20-DAY PROGRAM: YELLOW

Each of these sub-20-minute workouts is designed to help you build strength, stamina, and steely determination for the more advanced workouts in the orange and blue programs. You'll rotate through these workouts as indicated on the calendar, never doing the same workout twice in a row.

DOUBLE TROUBLE | Focus: Functional Strength

The name for this workout comes from the fact that exercises are done in superset fashion—two exercises done back-to-back without rest. The biggest benefit of this type of training method is that while one muscle group works, the other rests and vice versa. For example, when you do a superset that calls for a minute of squats followed immediately by a minute of push-ups, you are working two non-related muscle groups. As your chest and shoulders and triceps feel the burn on the push-ups, your legs get a bit of a break. This allows you to train at higher intensities throughout the workout.

You'll perform three supersets of two exercises, working each exercise for a minute straight, for a total of two rounds.

30 HI—30 LO | Focus: High Intensity Interval Training

This is the very definition of high intensity. You're going to give all you've got for 30 seconds straight, then you're going to rest and recover for 30 seconds before dialing it up again. These short bursts of all-out work are the absolute best way to build and cultivate metabolic muscle.

You'll perform five exercises for 30 seconds straight, resting 30 seconds between exercises, for a total of four rounds.

4x4 | Focus: Cardio Strength

Four exercises done consecutively without rest. By keeping rest to a minimum and forcing your body to work through several different moves in circuit fashion, you work a ton of muscle and scorch a boatload of calories in the process. But since the work periods are relatively short, you can still work each exercise at a very high level of effort.

You'll perform four exercises for a minute each, with no rest between exercises. You'll rest 1 minute between circuits and start from the top, running through the entire circuit four times total.

DOUBLE TROUBLE

Perform each superset twice. In each superset, you'll perform the two exercises listed for a minute each, back-to-back without rest. Rest 1 minute at the end of the superset and perform it once more before moving on to the next superset. Repeat the process with the next two supersets.

Superset 1:
1. Band Squat
2. Push-up

Superset 2:
1. Single-Leg Band Deadlift
2. Jumping Jacks

Superset 3:
1. Forearm Plank on Toes
2. Cobra-T

BAND SQUAT: Step on the band with feet shoulder width apart. Hold the band in each hand with palms facing each other at shoulder level.

Inhale as you bend your knees and push your hips behind your heels. Squat down until your thighs are parallel to the floor with your hips at knee level, keeping your hands at shoulder height and chest lifted.

Exhale and press through your heels as you return to the starting position.

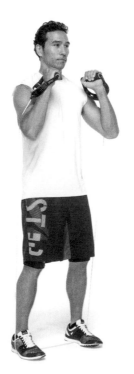
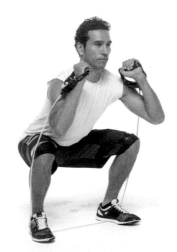

For the dumbbell version, hold a dumbbell in each hand at shoulder level with the dumbbells parallel to the floor, palms facing each other, and knuckles pointing toward the ceiling (this is a front-loaded movement). Perform reps as described for the band squat.

PUSH-UP: Start on your hands and toes in a plank position.

Inhale as you bend your arms to lower your body toward the ground. Lower yourself until your "belt buckle" and chest are a few inches off the ground before you push your body up to the starting position.

Exhale as you tighten your thighs and core, and push up to the starting position.

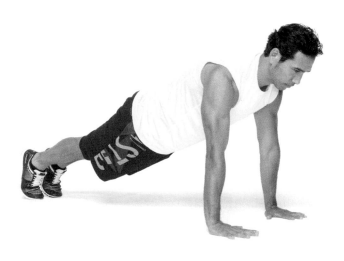

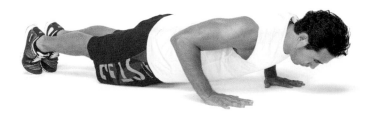

SINGLE-LEG BAND DEADLIFT: Loop the band in a big loop around your foot and place your foot where the band crosses. It should have enough resistance that it is difficult to pick up. Stand up and hold the band by the handles with a neutral grip (palms facing each other), arms at your sides.

Inhale as you bend your left knee slightly and push your hips behind your heels while lifting your right leg straight behind you. At the same time, bow forward with your chest lifted, back flat, and eyes on the floor. Your torso and rear right leg should end up parallel to the floor with toes pointing down. Then exhale as you press your left heel on the floor to return to the starting position with chest lifted. Alternate sides on each repetition.

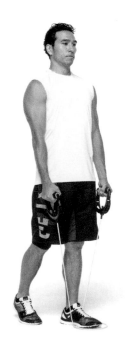
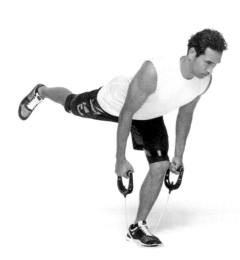

JUMPING JACKS: Start in a standing position with arms at sides.

Inhale as you jump your legs out to the sides while bringing your arms above your head.

Exhale and return to starting position and repeat for time.

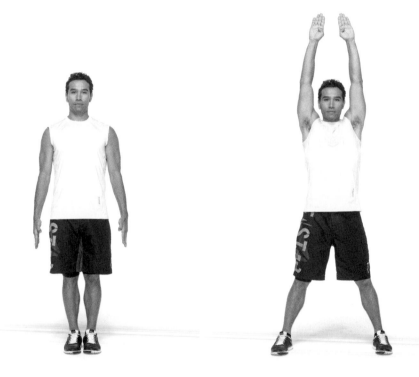

STRENGTH AND INSTABILITY

Testing your body's stability is a great way to build strength and balance. However, as instability goes up in an exercise, strength and power will go down. So you might find you need to use less weight for a one-legged version of a deadlift-row than for the two-legged version. Overall, you're going to get a bigger metabolic hit (in other words, your body has to work harder) and gain more strength from the moves that provide more stability. But by all means, try making exercises less stable to challenge yourself. Just know that there's a little bit of a trade-off in how much energy you'll be burning during those particular exercises.

FOREARM PLANK: Lie facedown on the floor with your forearms on floor parallel, palms facing down and elbows along your sides.

Exhale as you tighten your thighs and core while lifting yourself onto the balls of your feet with shoulders stacked above elbows and chin aligned just behind your wrists. Hold for time without holding your breath.

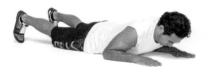 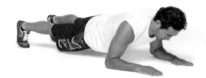

COBRA-T: Lie facedown on the floor with toes pointed, palms on the floor with hands underneath the shoulders, and elbows bent along your sides.

Squeeze your thighs so that your knees lift off the ground while drawing your shoulder blades together to lift your elbows slightly. Exhale as you take your hands off the ground and straighten your arms out to your sides in a T position while squeezing your lower, middle, and upper back to lift your upper body off the floor. Hold for time without holding your breath.

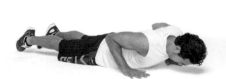 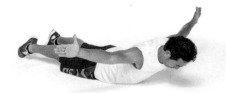

SCALE IT

Use these versions of the listed exercises to change the degree of difficulty.

SQUAT: To scale this down, simply ditch the band or dumbbell and use only your bodyweight. For a more advanced version, include an overhead press at the top with your palms facing forward and arms in line with your ears, or create a loop with the band to shorten it, thereby increasing tension.

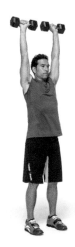

PUSH-UP: If you can't do regular push-ups, go from your knees while keeping your thighs, hips, and torso in a straight line. Allow your "belt buckle" and chest to come close to the floor at the same time when lowering yourself. If you can complete push-ups for a full minute, try Spiderman push-ups. When lowering yourself toward the floor, lift one leg off the ground and bend the knee toward your armpit in a "Spiderman" movement. Alternate sides each rep.

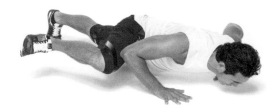

SINGLE-LEG DEADLIFT: Make this move easier by doing the one-leg, one-arm version without added resistance. Inhale as you bend forward at the waist and balance on your left leg as you bring your right leg up behind you, and your left arm up in front of you, in line with your torso. Exhale as you press your left heel on the floor and squeeze the back of your thighs and glutes to return to the starting position with chest lifted. Alternate sides on each repetition. To spice it up a bit, shorten the length of the band to increase resistance.

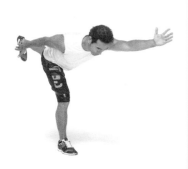

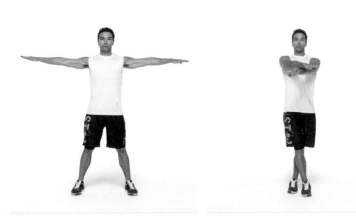

JUMPING JACKS: Can't handle the impact? Keep the same arm motion but "step out," one leg at a time and keep a brisk pace. To go more advanced, try the crossover jack, where you cross your arms above and below each other parallel to the floor in front of you while crossing your feet in front and behind each other on each rep.

FOREARM PLANK ON TOES: As with the push-up, you can make this move more tolerable by dropping your knees to the floor. For a tougher plank, pick one foot up off the ground with your leg straight and heel lifted (switch sides after 30 seconds).

COBRA-T: Make this move easier by keeping your arms in the starting position and lightly lifting your hands off the floor. For a tougher cobra, as you lift up, bend your elbows at 90 degrees with hands in front of you, thumbs pointing up, so that your arms make a W with your body.

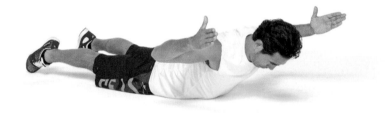

THE 4x4

Perform each of the four exercises listed for 1 minute, without resting between exercises, then rest 1 minute after completing the fourth exercise to make up one 5-minute round. Repeat the entire four-exercise sequence with the 1-minute rest three more times for a total of four, 5-minute rounds.

1. Dumbbell Stationary Lunge (30 seconds per side)
2. Band Row
3. Alternating 1-Leg Booty Bridge-V
4. Striders

DUMBBELL STATIONARY LUNGE: Start in a standing lunge position with left leg forward and one dumbbell in each hand with palms facing each other at shoulder height.

Inhale as you step forward and bend both knees to 90 degrees until your back knee is close to the floor with your chest lifted and eyes on the horizon.

Exhale as you press both feet into the floor to return to the starting position.

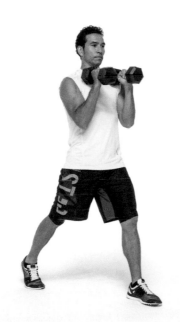 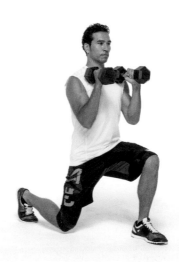

BAND ROW: Stand with feet shoulder distance apart, with weights in each hand; or step on the exercise band, holding one handle with each hand. Bend your knees and sit back slightly as you bow forward, hinging at the waist, until your chest is close to your thighs with your back flat, chin tucked, and eyes looking down. Your hands should be at knee level in a neutral grip (palms facing each other).

Exhale as you squeeze your shoulder blades together while pulling the handles toward your armpits, keeping your elbows along your ribs.

Inhale as you return your arms back toward your knees.

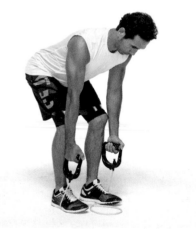 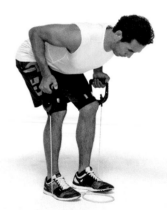

For the dumbbell version, use the same start position.

ALTERNATING 1-LEG BOOTY BRIDGE-V: Lie on your back with knees bent, feet on the floor directly under your knees hip distance apart, and arms low at your side in a V with your palms facing up.

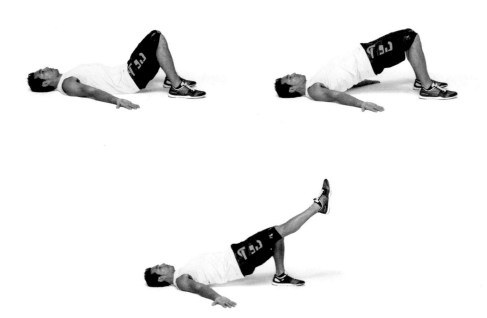

Inhale as you perform a booty bridge by pressing your heels into the floor and squeezing your glutes to lift your hips just below knee level.

In the raised position, exhale and lift one leg off the ground, extending it forward until it is straight, while keeping the thighs parallel.

Keeping your hips raised, inhale as your return your leg to the starting position and alternate extending your other leg. Take care not to twist or drop your hips—picture a glass of water being balanced on your belt buckle.

STRIDERS: Start in a standing lunge position with left leg forward and right arm forward. If possible, pick two spots on the floor (one near your left leg in the forward position and one near your right leg in the backward position) that you can use to "spot" the length of your lunge so that you don't jump too far, or not far enough, as you perform this movement.

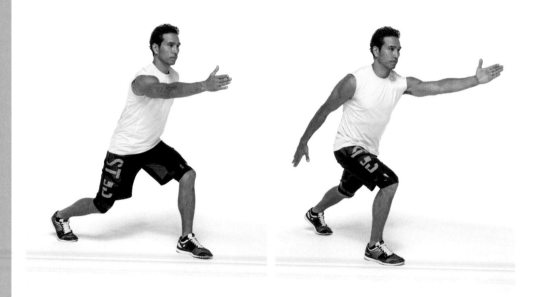

Exhale as you jump into a lunge position with right leg forward and left leg backward, moving your arms in tandem with your legs (right leg and left arm forward at the same time, and left leg and right arm forward at the same time).

Reverse the movement quickly. One key to this movement is to use your arms to drive your legs. Another key is not to jump too high; jump just enough to allow your feet to switch lunge positions.

SCALE IT

Use these versions of the listed exercises to change the degree of difficulty.

STATIONARY LUNGE: For an easier version, drop or lose the resistance. To make it more demanding, keep the resistance and add an overhead press at the top of each rep.

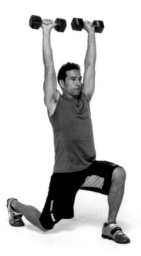

BAND ROW: For a slightly easier version, lower the resistance of the band or, if using dumbbells, use lighter weight. You can go more advanced by simply adding weight or alternating sides, pulling up with one side at a time.

ALTERNATING 1-LEG BOOTY BRIDGE-V: A basic booty bridge, with your arms in a T position on the floor, can be used if this version is too difficult. Or you can intensify the listed version by simply picking up your toes and shifting your weight onto your heels.

STRIDERS: You can scale down this exercise by performing toe tappers, where you simply alternate tapping your toes six inches in front of you and back, on the balls of your feet, for speed. Want to step it up? Clench your hands in fists and turn up the pace!

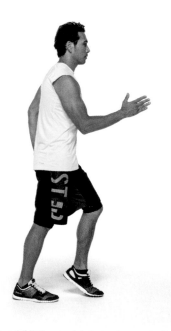
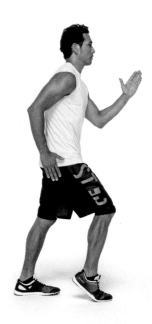

30 HI–30 LO

Perform each exercise listed for 30 seconds and rest for 30 seconds before moving on to the next exercise. It will take 5 minutes to complete
one five-exercise circuit. Perform four continuous circuits for a total of
20 minutes.

    1. Squat Thrust

    2. Jump Squat

    3. Push-Up-T (hands walk out-in)

    4. Run in Place

    5. Low-Hi Plank

SQUAT THRUST: Start in a standing position with legs shoulder width apart.

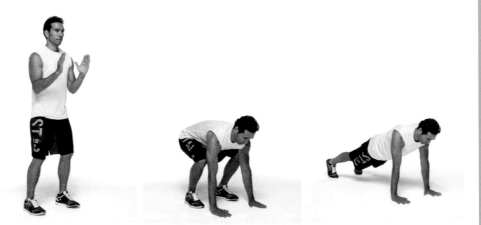

Inhale as you bend down and put your hands on the floor in front of your feet.

Exhale as you jump your legs behind you to a plank position while tightening your
core.

Inhale as you jump to bring your feet back toward your hands with both feet flat on
the floor, chest up, and eyes on the horizon. Exhale as you stand up and return to the
starting position.

JUMP SQUAT: Stand with your feet shoulder width apart, hands close to your chest.

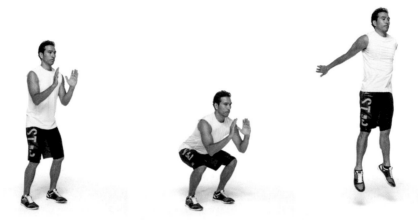

Inhale as you lower yourself down into the bottom of the squat with hands near chest at shoulder level.

Exhale as you drive through your heels quickly and jump in the air with hands thrusting down and behind you.

Take care to land softly in a squat position (knees bent and feet shoulder width apart).

PUSH UP-T: Perform a push-up as explained earlier in the Double Trouble workout.

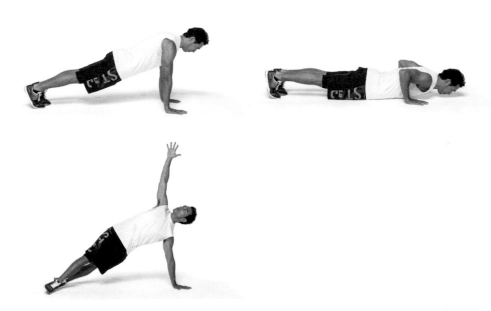

Then, turn your feet toe-to-heel and balance on your left arm as you move into a side plank and reach your right hand toward the ceiling so that your shoulders stack one on top of the other and your arms are in T position. Alternate sides with each rep.

RUN IN PLACE: Start by jogging in place and increase the pace of your steps so that you are running in place at a higher level of effort. The key to this exercise is keeping your elbows bent and having your arms drive your legs without your feet making much noise.

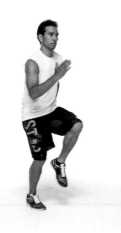

LOW-HI PLANK: Start in a basic plank position with your body straight and your arms extended with your palms flat on the floor. Inhale as you lower yourself to your forearms one at a time.

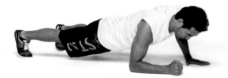
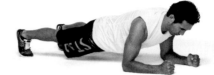

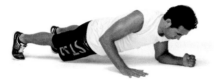

Then exhale and lift yourself back onto your palms, one at a time. Continue this motion for the allotted time.

SCALE IT

Use these versions of the listed exercises to change the degree of difficulty.

SQUAT THRUST: To take the explosive demands of this move down a notch, you can gently walk your legs out into the plank position and carefully walk them back in. Safe, continuous movement is key. For an added challenge, add in a push-up at the plank position and jump up as you come out of the squat position.

JUMP SQUAT: For a less explosive version, just do regular unweighted squats at as fast a pace as you can safely sustain for 30 seconds. If regular jump squats are too easy, try prisoner jump squats, where you keep your hands laced behind your head through each rep.

PUSH-UP-T: As with the regular push-up, you can get many of the same benefits by simply dropping to your knees and performing reps for the time allotted. To make the standard version harder, when you are in the side plank position, lift the top leg off your bottom leg to create a star shape with your body. Alternate sides each rep.

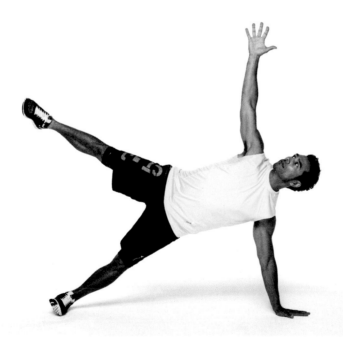

RUN IN PLACE: This one is easy to scale up or scale down. You can start at a comfortable pace and range of motion and work your way up to full-on, high-knee running.

LOW-HI PLANK: You can start from your knees to make the low-hi plank a bit easier or you can crank it up by lifting one hand off the ground in the "hi" position. Make sure you engage your thighs and core when lifting your hand so that your hips do not rotate. Then lower yourself and alternate hands each rep.

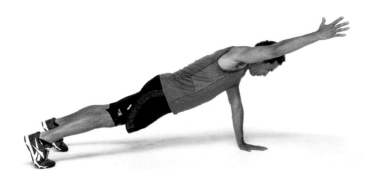

BPS: BODY-PART SPECIFIC

You'll perform supersets—two exercises back-to-back—each for a minute. Then you'll rest 30 seconds and move to the next superset. Repeat this for the second superset listed, then move on to the third superset.

Target: Booty
1. Alternating 1-Leg Booty Bridge-V
2. Capoeira Booty Kick (30 seconds per side)

Target: Chest (complete twice)
1. Band Chest Fly or Dumbbell Chest Fly Booty Bridge
2. Band Push-Up

Target: Abs

    1. Capoeira Knee Tuck Sit-Up

    2. Abs Leg Drop

ALTERNATING 1-LEG BOOTY BRIDGE-V: Perform a basic booty bridge as explained in the 4x4 workout.

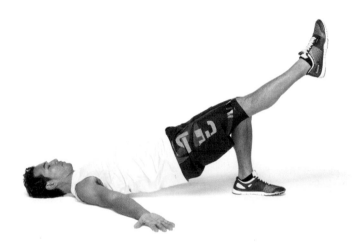

In the raised position, exhale and lift one leg off the ground, extending it forward until it is straight, while keeping the thighs parallel.

Keeping your hips raised, inhale as you return your leg to the starting position and alternate extending your other leg. Take care not to twist or drop your hips—picture a glass of water being balanced on your belt buckle.

CAPOEIRA BOOTY KICKS: Start on all fours on the floor with hands under shoulders and knees bent under hips.

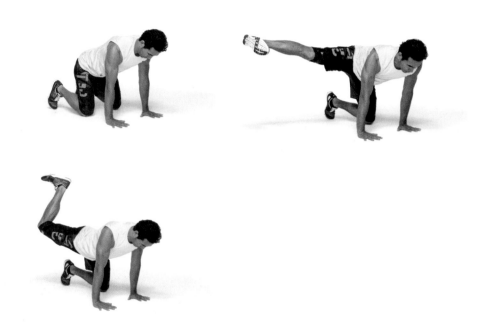

Exhale and raise your right leg to the side with your knee bent at 90 degrees and perform a roundhouse kick by straightening your right leg (think of trying to hit a target out to your side with your shoelaces).

Inhale and bring your knee back underneath your hips, then exhale and perform a donkey kick by pressing your heel back and up toward the ceiling with your knee bent at 90 degrees.

Return to starting position and reverse on the other side after 30 seconds.

BAND CHEST FLY: Begin in a lunge position with left leg forward and right leg behind you. Hold the handles of the exercise band with your arms extended to each side, stepping on the band with your right leg. Face your palms forward.

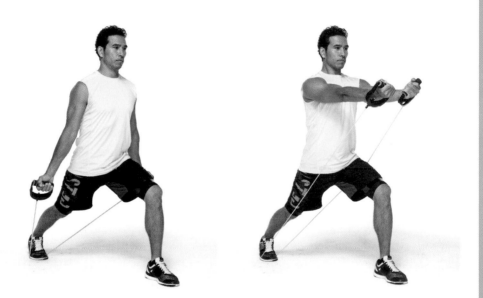

Exhale as you slowly move your arms forward in a wide arc, stopping just before your palms touch in front of you at your nipple line. Picture yourself driving your elbows and palms toward each other at the top of the movement.

Reverse the motion and repeat for reps.

DUMBBELL CHEST FLY BOOTY BRIDGE: Position yourself in a stable booty bridge position holding a pair of dumbbells out at your sides with your arms in a T and a slight bend in your elbows.

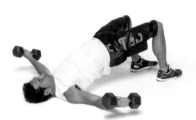 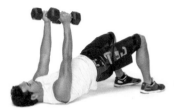

Exhale as you move the dumbbells up in a wide arc until they touch, then inhale as you slowly return them to the start position.

BAND PUSH-UP: Start in a kneeling position. Cross the band around your back and under your armpits. Use your right hand to hold the left side of the band and your left hand to hold the right side of the band so that the band makes an X at your chest.

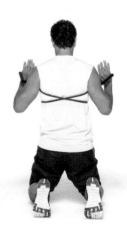 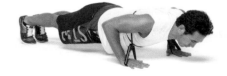

Get into a push-up position with your palms on the band.

For more tension, loop the band around your hands on each side. Perform the push-up in this position.

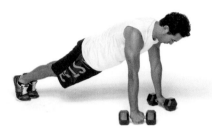 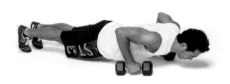

If using dumbbells, position the handles at a slight angle on the ground. Think of pointing your knuckles to the ground. Note that the dumbbell needs to be large enough for you to get your hands around it without touching the floor (an 8-pound or larger dumbbell should work). Perform the push-up holding the dumbbells.

CAPOEIRA KNEE TUCK SIT-UP: Lie on your back with your fists at your chest. Bend your knees and place your feet on the floor.

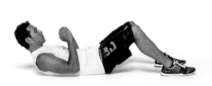 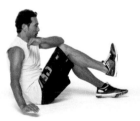

Inhale as you sit up, drawing your left knee into your chest, keeping your foot flexed and hands up.

Exhale as you return to the starting position. Repeat on your right side.

AB LEG DROP: Start by lying on your back with your hands laced behind your head, shoulder blades slightly lifted off the floor, chin tucked, eyes looking toward your "belt buckle," and both legs extended straight up to the ceiling.

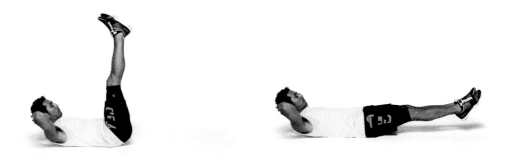

Inhale as you lower both legs until they are several inches off the ground and exhale as you lift your legs up to the starting position. The key to this exercise is keeping your back pressed flat against the floor and chin tucked.

SCALE IT

Use these versions of the listed exercises to change the degree of difficulty.

ALTERNATING BOOTY BRIDGE-V: A basic booty bridge, with your arms in a T position on the floor, can be used if this version is too difficult. Or you can enhance the listed version by simply picking up your toes and shifting your weight onto your heels, while alternating legs.

CAPOEIRA BOOTY KICKS: A more basic version of this move calls for you to raise your right leg to the side with your knee bent at 90 degrees until it is parallel to the floor, but not to perform the roundhouse kick. Then, perform a donkey kick by pressing your heel back and up toward the ceiling with your knee bent at 90 degrees. Do this for 30 seconds, then switch to the other side. Need to go more advanced? Try the capoeira half-moon booty kick. In this variation, take your right leg and touch your toe as far forward as you can out to your right side, then trace your foot all the way behind you and up in a half-moon shape by leading with your heel. Do this for 30 seconds, then switch to the other side.

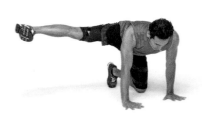 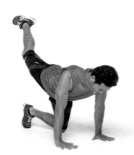

BAND CHEST FLY: If the weighted version is too challenging, scale down by simply performing a wide push-up from the knees. To make it more advanced, step on a band with your back foot, arms at side, palms facing forward. Bring your arms forward to chest level, palms facing in. Add a short pulse rep after you bring palms together. To increase the demand with dumbbells, lie on your back with your hips bridged up off the floor, weight on your heels, arms out to your sides with a slight bend in elbows, palms facing up. When your arms are apart at the bottom, add a short pulse rep before lifting arms in a wide arc to top.

BAND PUSH-UP: For a lighter version, ditch the band or dumbbell and do a body-weight push-up on your knees. At the bottom of each rep, allow your body to touch the floor, then pick your hands up off the floor before placing them back down and pushing yourself back up from the floor. A more advanced version calls for you to perform the push-up on your toes, with 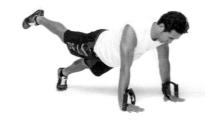 the band or the dumbbell, but to pick one leg up off the floor on each rep, being careful to keep your core stable throughout.

CAPOEIRA KNEE TUCK SIT-UP: For an easier version that hits the same muscles, try the capoeira sit-up punch, where you sit up until your chest is close to your knees and then punch diagonally across the body with each hand.

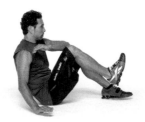 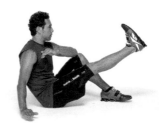

More advanced individuals can try the **Capoeira Push-Kick Sit-Up (*Bênção* Sit-Up)**. As you perform the sit-up, draw your left knee into your chest. Keep your foot flexed and your hands up. Then, push your left leg out in front of you, leading with your heel, and sweep your right arm across your chest with elbow bent. Your left arm will extend to the left side. Return to starting position and repeat on the other side.

AB LEG DROP: If you're new to this move, or if your lower back begins to fatigue, try it with bent knees.

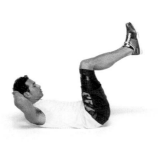 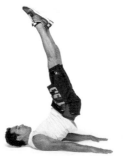

To increase the demand on your abs, thrust your legs and "belt buckle" toward the ceiling after you lift them up on each rep. Your hips should lift off the ground with your legs staying in the same vertical line.

BUSTING THROUGH PLATEAUS

There comes a time when you need to introduce your body to new challenges—to break new barriers. Twenty days is a great base to build from, but it is also around the time that your body starts to get used to what you're putting it through. *And that's a bad thing*, because when your body gets used to the same workouts week in and week out, something strange happens—it stops getting stronger, it stops releasing fat, and it stops making progress. It figures, "Okay, well, I finally caught up to what she was asking of me, so I can kick back for a while now!"

This is called hitting a plateau and it happens to everyone . . . unless you change things up. And that's where the orange and blue programs come in—two additional 20-day programs that you can use to take your training to the next level. You don't want your body to ever get too comfortable!

Exercises can be made harder by altering any one (or more) of the following variables:

1. RESISTANCE. Add resistance in the form of dumbbells or an exercise band. Increase resistance as the exercise gets easier. Once you can do more reps than are being asked of you for a given exercise or across a given time period, it's time to step things up. And don't be afraid to lift weights that are challenging. "Heavy" is relative and you're not likely to bulk up (I'm looking at you, ladies) from using heavier loads. You're also not likely to change your body if you use the same weights all the time.

2. INSTABILITY. Try a movement on one leg if it's a standing movement, or on one arm if it's an arm movement (like a one-armed plank). When one side of your body has to work extra hard, you're really challenging yourself to improve rapidly by engaging more of the small, stabilizer muscles throughout your body that work overtime to make the micro-corrections necessary to keep you balanced.

3. REPETITIONS. Try doing more repetitions (be sure to keep good form) per exercise. If you could do five push-ups earlier this week in a workout, try for six in the next workout. Did 15 reps in a minute today? Great. Try for 16 or more next time, or increase the weight (see No. 1).

4. SPEED. If the exercise warrants it, try performing the exercise more quickly. The faster you move, the harder that exercise becomes. Just remember to use good form and you'll get more out of a faster movement.

20-DAY FITNESS PLAN: ORANGE

It's a pretty great thing to discover the value of training hard for 20 minutes and calling it quits. The workouts in the orange program use the same time constraints but pack an even greater punch because of the unique, high intensity schemes that I've devised for you.

Before each workout, you'll perform a short, active warm-up (see pages 90–91) to prep your body and nervous system for the work to come.

THE 20-DAY CALENDAR: ORANGE

In the orange program, you'll borrow a few of the protocols that you followed in the yellow program, including the 30 HI–30 LO and the 4x4. The 30 HI–30 LO and 4x4 get small upgrades (Version 2), but taking the place of Double Trouble workouts will be the Triple Threat, which ups the ante enough to coax your body into torching even more fat!

DAY	WORKOUT/ACTIVITY
1	Triple Threat
2	4x4 Version 2
3	30 HI–30 LO Version 2
4	Rest, Body-Part Specific or Cardio-Air
5	Triple Threat
6	4x4 Version 2
7	Rest
8	Triple Threat
9	4x4 Version 2
10	30 HI–30 LO Version 2
11	Rest, Body-Part Specific or Cardio-Air
12	Triple Threat
13	30 HI–30 LO Version 2
14	Rest
15	Triple Threat

16	4x4 Version 2
17	30 HI–30 LO Version 2
18	Rest, Body-Part Specific or Cardio-Air
19	4x4 Version 2
20	30 HI–30 LO Version 2

On Days 4, 11, and 18, you have the option to perform a body-part specific (BPS) or cardio-air workout.

THE 20-DAY PROGRAM: ORANGE

The Orange program is a step up from what you did with the yellow program. Each of these sub-20-minute workouts holds something different for you. Mixing it up from day to day ensures that your body is always off balance, which is the key to avoiding plateaus.

TRIPLE THREAT | Focus: Functional Strength

The yellow Double Trouble workouts introduced you to the concept of supersets—two exercises done in a row without rest. Now, you're going to do trisets—three exercises done back-to-back-to-back without rest. This challenges your muscular strength and endurance and also has the benefit of burning additional calories in the workout because the work is condensed. The increased demand on your muscles also means greater post-workout calorie burn.

You'll perform three exercises in a row for 1 minute each. Rest 1 minute, then repeat the triset. Rest 1 minute, then repeat the process with the second triset listed.

30 HI–30 LO VERSION 2 | Focus: High Intensity Interval Training

This is the very definition of high intensity. You're going to give all you've got for 30 seconds straight, then you're going to rest and recover for 30 seconds before dialing it up again. These short bursts of all-out work are the absolute best way to build and cultivate metabolic muscle.

You'll perform five exercises for 30 seconds straight, resting 30 seconds between exercises, for a total of four rounds.

4x4 VERSION 2 | Focus: Cardio Strength

Four exercises done consecutively without rest. By keeping rest to a minimum and forcing your body to work through several different moves in circuit fashion, you work a ton of muscle and scorch a boatload of calories in the process. But since the work periods are relatively short, you can still work each exercise at a very high level of effort.

You'll perform four exercises for a minute each, with no rest between exercises. You'll rest 1 minute between circuits and start from the top, running through the entire circuit four times.

BODY-PART SPECIFIC | Focus: Individual Muscle Groups

The three main workouts in this program are designed to work your entire body. But, if you're up for it, on Days 4, 11, and 18, you can perform a body-part specific workout where you target individual muscles—like your butt or your abs—for additional work. The cost of your additional work is low: these workouts can be completed in about 7 minutes.

You'll perform two exercises back-to-back, each for a minute. Then you'll rest 30 seconds and move to the next superset. Repeat this for the second superset listed, then move on to the third superset.

CARDIO-AIR | Focus: Additional Calorie Burn

The only break I'll give you from metabolic muscle workouts is completely optional. You will do just fine on your program without these cardio-air workouts, but if you're really itching to move, I'm not going to discourage you too much. You *may* use your optional days to do 30–60 minutes of select cardio activities at a moderate pace. These workouts will help you burn a few additional calories, but they don't trigger the afterburn that we're going for. My eight suggested options for this workout are treadmill, elliptical, rower, recumbent bike, boxing/kickboxing, swimming, VersaClimber, and dance class, but other similar activities are certainly acceptable. Less experienced individuals can get away with a lighter pace on these activities, while more experienced individuals can increase intensity at their discretion. Again, this workout is entirely optional.

You'll perform one of the cardio-based activities listed at a moderate but consistent pace for 30–60 minutes.

TRIPLE THREAT

You'll perform three exercises in a row for 1 minute each. Rest 1 minute at the end of the triset, then repeat the triset. Continue this process with the second triset listed.

Triset 1:
1. Band Thruster
2. Dumbbell $\frac{1}{2}$ Hoebel Curl
3. Jump Switch Punches

Triset 2:

    1. 1-Leg Deadlift with Knee Lift with Band (30 seconds per side)

    2. Cross-Over Plank

    3. Alternating 1-Leg Booty Bridge-V

BAND THRUSTER: Stand with legs hip distance apart, holding dumbbells or band in a neutral grip (palms facing each other) at shoulder level. This movement is a squat combined with an overhead press.

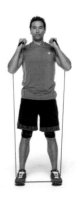 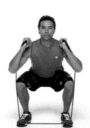 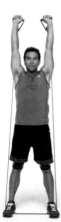

Inhale as you squat down until your thighs are parallel to the floor with hips at knee level, keeping your hands at shoulder height and your chest lifted.

Exhale as you push through your heels to stand up and press the dumbbells or band handles overhead with palms facing forward and arms in line with ears.

Return to starting position.

DUMBBELL ½ HOEBEL CURL: With your palms in a neutral grip, perform a curl.

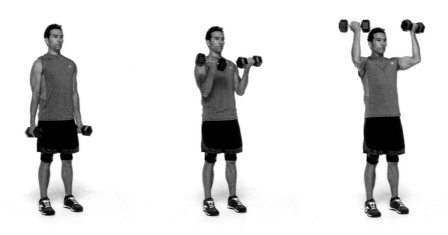

At the top of the movement, elevate your shoulders while keeping your elbows bent at 90 degrees until your elbows are even with your shoulders, upper arms parallel to the floor. Return to the starting position.

If using a band, stand on the band with feet shoulder width apart, with your palms in a neutral grip. Inhale as you perform a curl and bring your hands close to your shoulders. At the top of the curl, exhale as you raise your elbows to shoulder level, keeping your arms bent at 90 degrees with palms facing you. Return to the starting position.

JUMP SWITCH PUNCHES: Get into a staggered stance with left leg forward and right leg back, and with fists below your chin, palms facing each other. Alternate punching in front of you with both hands in a staggered rhythm (left, right, then repeat).

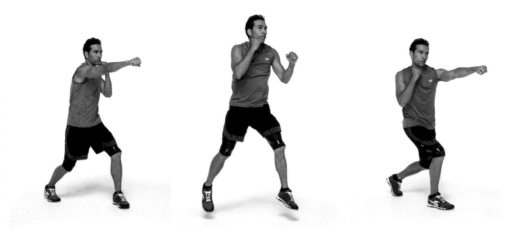

Switch your foot position by performing a small jump (lifting both feet off the floor) every few seconds

1-LEG DEADLIFT KNEE LIFT WITH BAND: Loop the band in a big loop around your foot and place your foot where the band crosses. It should have enough resistance that it is difficult to pick up.

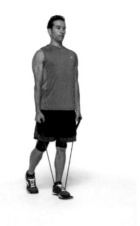

Stand up and hold the band by the handles with a neutral grip (palms facing each other), arms at your sides.

Inhale as you bend your left knee slightly and push your hips behind your heels while lifting your right leg straight behind you.

At the same time, bow forward with your chest lifted, back flat, and eyes on the floor.

Your torso and rear right leg should end up parallel to the floor with toes pointing down.

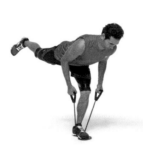 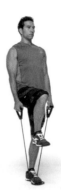

Then, exhale as you press your left heel on the floor and pull your right knee through to the front of your body up to hip level before returning to the starting position with chest lifted.

For variety, you can perform the 1-leg deadlift with knee lift holding dumb-bells in a neutral grip at your sides.

CROSS-OVER PLANK: Start in plank position.

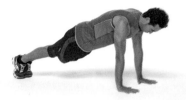 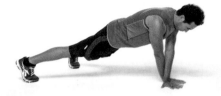

Move to the right by stepping your right foot farther out to the right while crossing your left hand over your right hand.

Keep moving to the right by stepping your left foot to the right while moving your right hand to the right so that you end up in a plank position again. Repeat the movement to the opposite side.

ALTERNATING 1-LEG BOOTY BRIDGE-V: Lie on your back with knees bent, feet on the floor directly under your knees hip distance apart, and arms at your side in a V with your palms facing up.

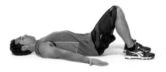 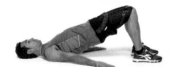

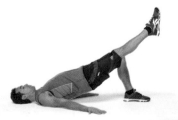

Inhale as you perform a booty bridge by pressing your heels into the floor and squeezing your glutes to lift your hips just below knee level.

In the raised position, exhale and lift one leg off the ground, extending it forward until it is straight, while keeping the thighs parallel.

Keeping your hips raised, inhale as your return your leg to the starting position and alternate extending your other leg. Take care not to twist or drop your hips—picture a glass of water being balanced on your belt buckle.

SCALE IT

Use these versions of the listed exercises to change the degree of difficulty.

BAND THRUSTER: If thrusters are too challenging, you can lighten the resistance or substitute basic bodyweight squats. To make it tougher, add a small jump at the top of the thruster.

DUMBBELL ½ HOEBEL CURL: Standard curls will suffice if this version is too tough to do for time. If the minute is too easy, simply add to the resistance you're using or, with the same weight, try to get more reps in the given time.

JUMP SWITCH PUNCHES: To simmer this one down, you can just carefully "walk" your feet into position instead of jumping. To increase the difficulty, perform a higher jump as you switch your feet.

1-LEG DEADLIFT WITH KNEE LIFT: For an easier version, skip the knee lift on each rep. To make it harder, you can add a row on one leg when your torso is parallel to the floor, then stand straight up again and add a knee lift at the top of the movement. For this exercise, if you are using an exercise band, fold the band in half and step on it to create resistance.

CROSS-OVER PLANK: Do this from your knees if you can't make it with the listed version for a full minute. To go more advanced, perform the same movement from your toes but after moving to the right, kick your right leg out to the side before reversing the movement. Engage your core to prevent your hips from rotating during the kick. After moving to the left, kick the left leg out to the side.

ALTERNATING 1-LEG BOOTY BRIDGE-V: The booty bridge with your arms in a T position on the floor will suffice if the listed version is too tough to sustain for a minute straight. Need a scaled-up variation? Try the 1-leg booty bridge knee tuck on your heels with a band or dumbbell. With the band variation, you'll place your feet in the band handles and pull the band over your hips with knees bent. Keep the knee of the resting leg tucked into your chest. Do this for 30 seconds, then switch to the other side. To add more resistance, loop the band around each foot before pulling the band over your hips.

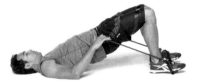 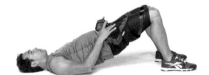

For the dumbbell variation, balance a dumbbell below your belly button during the movement and hold with one hand to keep balanced. Do this for 30 seconds, then switch to the other side.

THE 4x4 VERSION 2

Perform each of the four exercises listed for 1 minute to make up one 4-minute round. Rest 1 minute. Then, repeat the entire four-exercise sequence three more times for a total of four 4-minute rounds.

1. Capoeira Reverse Lunge (*Decida Básica*) (30 seconds per side)
2. Wide-Grip Band Row

3. Alternating 1-Leg Booty Bridge-W

4. Cheerleaders

CAPOEIRA REVERSE LUNGE (*DECIDA BÁSICA*): *Decida Básica* means a "basic descent" and is a defensive move in capoeira to duck an attack. Start in a standing position with legs shoulder width apart.

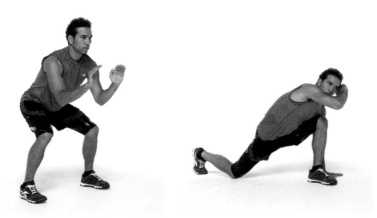

Inhale as you step back with your right leg into a low lunge until both knees are bent at 90 degrees, with your left knee aligned above your left heel and your right knee just above the ground. Bring your left hand to the ground (palm flat on the floor), to the outside of your left foot with fingers pointing to the left. Your chest should be close to your left thigh and your head slightly tilted to the left as if you ducked a kick. Move your right elbow in front of your face, almost as though you're kissing your biceps—in capoeira, this is a move to protect your face.

Exhale as you press your right heel into the floor while engaging your core to return to the standing position. Perform the same movement on the other side, then continue alternating sides.

WIDE-GRIP ROW: Stand with feet shoulder-width apart, holding one weight in each hand. Bend your knees and sit back slightly as you bow forward, hinging at the waist, until your chest is close to your thighs with your back flat, chin tucked, and eyes looking down. Your hands will be at knee level in a pronated grip (palms facing your shins).

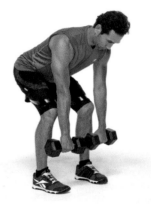 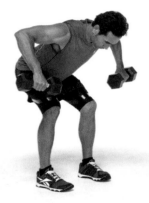

Exhale as you squeeze your shoulder blades together while pulling the weights up and out in a wide arc until your elbows are at shoulder level and bent at 90 degrees at the top of the movement.

Inhale as you return your arms back toward your knees.

ALTERNATING 1-LEG BOOTY BRIDGE-W: Lie on your back with knees bent, feet on the floor directly under your knees, hip distance apart. Extend your arms on the floor to either side in a W position with your elbows bent at 90 degrees and palms facing up. Make sure the back of your head and wrists press into the floor to engage your shoulder blades and upper back.

Inhale as you perform a booty bridge as explained in the Triple Threat workout.

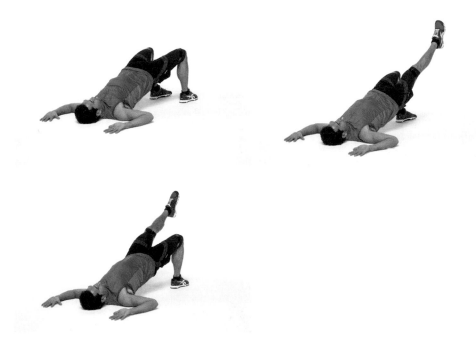

In the raised position, exhale and lift one leg off the ground, extending it forward until it is straight, while keeping the thighs parallel. Keeping your hips raised, inhale as you return your leg to the starting position and alternate extending your other leg. Take care not to twist or drop your hips—picture a glass of water being balanced on your belt buckle.

CHEERLEADERS: Begin in a standing position with your arms raised above your head.

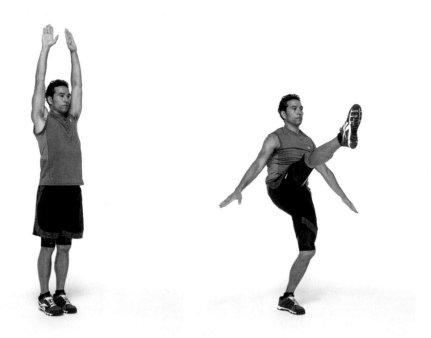

Exhale as you quickly pull your arms to your sides and kick your right leg forward and up to hip level or higher.

Inhale as you return your arms to the starting position. Repeat on the left side and continue alternating each rep.

SCALE IT

Use these versions of the listed exercises to change the degree of difficulty.

CAPOEIRA REVERSE LUNGE: An easier version is *Esquiva Normal*, which means a "normal escape" and is another defensive move in capoeira to duck an attack. It is basically a stationary lunge with a bow. Start in a standing lunge position with left leg forward.

Your left hand is by your left hip with palm facing down and fingers pointing to the left, and your right elbow is bent at 90 degrees in front of your face. Inhale as you lower your right knee toward the floor until it is just above the ground while bowing forward until your chest is close to your thigh with left hand close to the floor and head slightly tilted to the left as if you ducked a kick. Exhale as you press your feet into the ground to return to the starting position. Do this for 30 seconds, then repeat the on other side. For a more advanced version, perform a knee strike when coming up from the low lunge by pushing your right knee forward and up as you lean back. Your arms will switch as you do the knee strike and they will switch again as you return to the original standing lunge position. Do this for 30 seconds, then repeat on the other side.

WIDE-GRIP BAND ROW: To make this easier, perform it with a closer grip, where you start with your palms facing each other in a closer grip and your arms pull alongside you until your elbows are bent at 90 degrees. To make this a bit tougher, increase band resistance by making it shorter or alternate sides by pulling up with one side at a time.

ALTERNATING 1-LEG BOOTY BRIDGE-W: For a scaled-down version, do a booty bridge with your arms in a V. To step it up a notch, perform the W bridge and bring your toes off the ground to put all the weight on your heels (and all the stress on your booty!).

CHEERLEADERS: If this move is too difficult to master, try striders, where you basically switch your feet quickly front to back in a partial lunge (see the 4x4 workout in the yellow program for more details). To scale up, clench your fists in the cheerleader movement.

30 HI–30 LO VERSION 2

Perform each exercise listed for 30 seconds and rest for 30 seconds before moving on to the next exercise. It will take 5 minutes to complete one five-exercise circuit. Perform four continuous circuits for a total of 20 minutes.

1. Squat Thrust-Jump
2. Jump Squat with $\frac{1}{4}$ Turn

3. Push-Up Star

4. High Knees Running

5. Low-Hi Plank with 1-Hand Lift

SQUAT THRUST-JUMP: Start in a standing position with legs shoulder width apart.

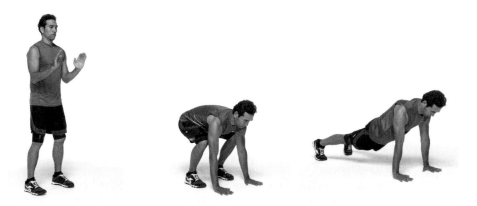

Inhale as you bend down and put your hands on the floor in front of your feet.

Exhale as you jump your legs behind you to a plank position while tightening your core.

Inhale as you jump to bring your feet back toward your hands with both feet flat on the floor, chest up, and eyes on the horizon. Exhale as you stand up and return to the starting position and jump in the air with your arms above your head.

JUMP SQUAT WITH ¼ TURN: Start in a standing position with feet shoulder width apart.

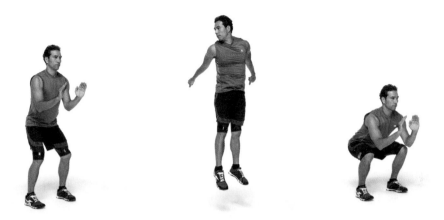

Perform a jump squat with a ¼ turn to the right while you are in the air.

Land facing your right.

Perform ¼ turn jump squats until you are facing forward again. Reverse the turns for the next set of four squats, jumping and turning to the left.

PUSH-UP STAR: Start in a regular push-up position. This is a cross between a push-up and a side plank with a leg raise.

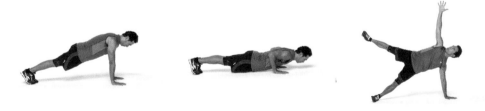

Perform the push-up, and then turn your feet toe to heel and balance on your left arm as you move into a side plank and reach your right hand upward. When you are in the side plank position, lift the top leg off your bottom leg to create a "star" shape with your body. Alternate sides for each rep.

20-DAY FITNESS PLAN: ORANGE

HIGH KNEES RUNNING: Simply run in place, bringing your knees high on every stride. Work up to the fastest pace you can sustain for 30 seconds.

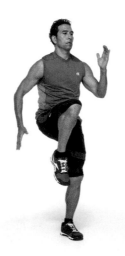
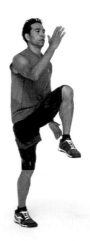

LO-HI PLANK WITH 1-HAND LIFT: Start in a basic plank position with your body straight and your arms extended with your palms flat on the floor.

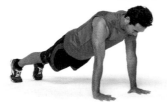
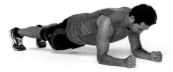

Inhale as you lower yourself to your forearms one at a time in the "low" position.

Then exhale as you lift yourself back onto your palms, one at a time, to the starting "high" position.

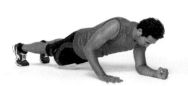 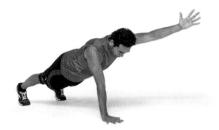

At the top of the movement, inhale as you lift one hand off the ground while engaging your thighs and core so that your hips do not rotate.

Exhale as you place your hand back on the floor to the starting position. Alternate lifting the opposite hand every rep and continue this "lo-hi" motion for the allotted time.

SCALE IT

Use these versions of the listed exercises to change the degree of difficulty.

SQUAT THRUST-JUMP: To scale this down a bit, "walk" your feet back into the plank position instead of "jumping" them back. To get more intense, add a sprawl by jumping back with your legs and lowering your body fully to the ground before jumping forward with your legs.

JUMP SQUAT WITH ¼ TURN: An easier variation involves doing a regular squat followed by a jump squat. To go harder, try the prisoner jump squat with ¼ turn by keeping your hands laced behind your head.

PUSH-UP STAR: If the star version keeps you from sustaining a good pace, revert back to the T position (no raising the leg). Want to get trickier? Try the "shooting star" version, where you walk your hands and feet out to the side and back before doing your push-up star. And if you still want more, try jumping your hands and feet instead of walking them.

HIGH KNEES RUNNING: You can easily slow your pace down if you need to lighten the intensity, but try to keep your knees coming to waist height on each stride. If you want to turn it up, after every eight strides add a tuck jump where you jump and tuck your knees up to your waist level in the air.

LO-HI PLANK WITH 1-HAND LIFT: As with most plank variations, you can try this one from your knees if you are fatiguing before 30 seconds. To scale it up, however, you can reach out in front of you with each hand at the top before lowering your body back to your elbows.

BPS: BODY-PART SPECIFIC

You'll perform two exercises back-to-back, each for a minute. Then you'll rest 30 seconds and move to the next superset. Repeat this for the second superset listed, then move on to the third superset.

Target: Booty
1. Alternating 1-Leg Booty Bridge-V on Heels
2. Capoeira Half-Moon Booty Kick (30 seconds per side)

Target: Chest
1. Push-Up with 1-Hand Lift
2. Traveling Push-Up

Target: Abs
1. Capoeira Sit-Up Plank
2. Alternating Abs Jackknife-Toe

ALTERNATING 1-LEG BOOTY BRIDGE-V ON HEELS: Perform the basic booty bridge on your heels.

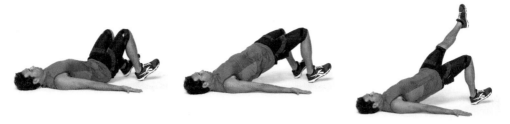

In the raised position, exhale and lift one leg off the ground, extending it forward until it is straight, while keeping the thighs parallel.

Keeping your hips raised, inhale as you return your leg to the starting position and alternate extending your other leg. Take care not to twist or drop your hips—picture a glass of water being balanced on your belt buckle.

CAPOEIRA HALF-MOON BOOTY KICK: Start on all fours on the floor with hands under shoulders and knees bent under hips.

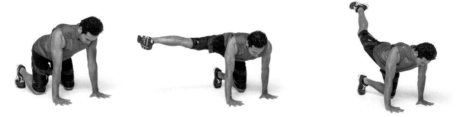

Inhale as you take your right leg and touch your toe as far forward as you can out to your right side.

Then exhale as you trace your foot all the way behind you and up in a half-moon shape by leading with your heel.

Do this for 30 seconds, then switch to the other side.

PUSH-UP WITH 1-HAND LIFT: Perform a push-up. At the top of the movement, lift one hand off the ground without allowing your hips to rotate.

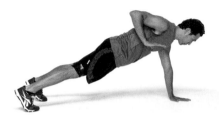

TRAVELING PUSH-UP: Perform a push-up.

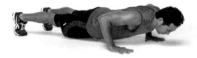

Move your hands and feet a step to the left, then perform a push-up in that position.

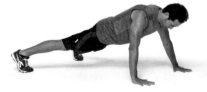
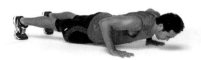

Move your hands and feet a step to your right, then perform a push-up. Repeat.

CAPOEIRA SIT-UP PLANK: Start lying on your back with knees up, heels on the ground, and hands in front of your chest, chin tucked, looking between your legs, and shoulder blades slightly lifted off the floor.

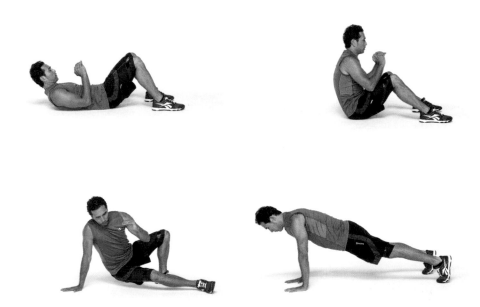

Exhale as you perform a sit-up by engaging your core and lifting your torso off the ground.

Inhale at the top of the sit-up and turn your body to the left to go into a plank position, balancing on your hands and toes.

Exhale as you turn back into the top of the sit-up position. Inhale as you return to the starting position on the ground. Perform the entire movement to the other side.

ALTERNATING ABS JACKKNIFE-TOE: Lie on your back with legs fully extended and arms extended above your head.

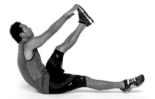

As you exhale, simultaneously lift your head/torso and your right leg. Reach for your toes with both arms.

Inhale as you lower your leg and torso. Repeat with your left leg.

SCALE IT

Use these versions of the listed exercises to change the degree of difficulty.

ALTERNATING 1-LEG BOOTY BRIDGE-V ON HEELS: To make it easier, keep your feet flat on the floor. For a slightly more difficult variation, perform a booty bridge, from the floor, with one leg on your heel for 30 straight seconds. Lift your free leg up straight until your thighs are parallel, then switch to the other side and repeat for 30 seconds.

CAPOEIRA HALF-MOON BOOTY KICK: If this is too difficult, try the capoeira booty kicks. This variation adds a roundhouse kick before you perform a donkey kick. Raise your right leg to the side with your knee bent at 90 degrees and perform a roundhouse kick by straightening your right leg (think of trying to hit a target out to your side with your shoelaces). Then

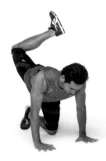

inhale and bring your knee back underneath your hips. Exhale and perform a donkey kick by pressing your heel back and up toward the ceiling with your knee bent at 90 degrees. Do this for 30 seconds, then reverse on the other side. A more advanced version is the Capoeira Scorpion Kick. To do it right, perform the half-moon kick out to the right side, toe on the ground, and then perform a scorpion kick by bringing your leg up and behind you, and bending your knee to make your right leg look like a scorpion's tail. Do this for 30 seconds, then reverse the movement on the other side.

PUSH-UP WITH 1-HAND LIFT: Any push-up variation is made easier by taking it to your knees. To make it harder, however, you can reach your arm straight out in front of you at the top of each rep.

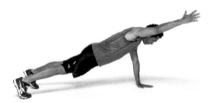

TRAVELING PUSH-UP: For an easier version, start from your knees. To scale up, lift one leg when performing the push-up to add an element of balance. This calls more stabilizer muscles into play, increasing your calorie burn. Alternate legs each rep.

CAPOEIRA SIT-UP PLANK: For a slightly easier variation, do the plank part of the movement on your knees instead of your toes. A tougher variation calls for a knee strike. When you flip to the plank position on your left side, quickly pull your right knee to your chest as a knee strike. Do the knee strike on the other side during the next rep.

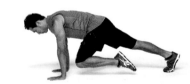

ALTERNATING ABS JACKKNIFE: If your toe is out of reach, your shin will do. To make it harder, lift both legs off the floor while performing the movement.

20-DAY FITNESS PLAN: BLUE

The next level. The next phase in your journey (there's never a last). The blue level represents the culmination of everything that you've worked so hard for over the course of the first two 20-day programs. The workouts are harder and your muscles and lungs will be screaming for mercy, but by now, you're battle-tested and capable of so much more than you were 40 days ago!

Before each workout, you'll perform a short, active warm-up (see pages 90–91) to prep your body and nervous system for the work to come.

THE 20-DAY CALENDAR: BLUE

In the blue program, there will be some familiar elements, but we're taking it to a whole new level with the introduction of the 100s workout. It's a notoriously tough cardio-strength workout and, yes, 100 is the number of reps you'll do per exercise. Prepare to sweat! You'll do "just" two exercises in this workout as a superset, for 10 rounds, which really puts working muscles to the test.

DAY	WORKOUT/ACTIVITY
1	Triple Threat
2	100s
3	30 HI–30 LO Version 3
4	Rest, Body-Part Specific or Cardio-Air
5	Triple Threat
6	100s
7	Rest
8	Triple Threat
9	100s
10	30 HI–30 LO Version 3
11	Rest, Body-Part Specific or Cardio-Air
12	Triple Threat

13	30 HI–30 LO Version 3
14	Rest
15	Triple Threat
16	100s
17	30 HI–30 LO Version 3
18	Rest, Body-Part Specific or Cardio-Air
19	100s
20	30 HI–30 LO Version 2

On Days 4, 11, and 18, you have the option to perform a body-part specific (BPS) or cardio-air workout.

THE 20-DAY PROGRAM: BLUE

TRIPLE THREAT | Focus: Functional Strength

Continuing with the triset approach—three exercises in a row—from the orange program, you will progress to more challenging, multi-joint movements. The exercises in this program challenge not only main movers like your legs, shoulders, and back but also the deeper, unseen muscles of your core that support your abs, enhance posture, and increase balance.

You'll perform three exercises in a row for 1 minute each. Rest 1 minute, then repeat the triset. Rest 1 minute, then repeat the process with the second triset listed.

100s | Focus: Strength, Endurance, Calorie Burn

The cornerstone of the blue program, the 100s workout calls for a very high volume of work in a very short period of time. Pairing two exercises back-to-back in a superset dials up the intensity, and then you throw fuel on the metabolic fire by performing this superset 10 times. The moves assigned are challenging but not impossible. The real task is maintaining solid form throughout the entire workout, so fatigue and mental toughness come into play as well.

You'll perform two exercises, back-to-back and without rest, before taking a 45-second break. You'll perform 10 total supersets.

30 HI–30 LO | Focus: High Intensity Interval Training

In terms of the sheer difficulty of the exercises, this may actually be the toughest of the blue workouts. The inclusion of more taxing exercises like star jumps and burpees, all done in high intensity interval fashion, definitely ups the physical ante of this retooled 30 HI–30 LO sweat session. The aim, once again, is to give everything you have for 30 straight seconds before taking a 30-second breather.

Perform each exercise listed for 30 seconds and rest for 30 seconds before moving on to the next exercise. It will take 5 minutes to complete one five-exercise circuit. Perform four continuous circuits for a total of 20 minutes.

BODY-PART SPECIFIC | Focus: Individual Muscle Groups

By this phase of your training, you are likely to have more energy, strength, and ambition. Why not use this to your advantage with a few extra, if optional, workouts? If you're up for it, on Days 4, 11, and 18, you can perform a body-part specific workout where you target individual muscles—like your butt or your abs—for additional work. The cost of your additional work is low: these workouts can be completed in about 7 minutes. This additional work can help bolster your already stellar gains.

You'll perform two exercises back-to-back, each for a minute. Then you'll rest 30 seconds and move to the next superset. Repeat this for the second superset listed, then move on to the third superset.

CARDIO-AIR | Focus: Additional Calorie Burn

As with the previous programs, you *may* use your optional days to do 30–60 minutes of select cardio activities at a moderate pace. These workouts will help you burn a few additional calories, but they don't trigger the afterburn that we're going for. My eight suggested options for this workout are treadmill, elliptical, rower, recumbent bike, boxing/kickboxing, swimming, VersaClimber, and dance class, but other similar activities are certainly acceptable. Less experienced individuals can get away with a lighter pace on these activities, while more experienced individuals can increase intensity at their discretion. Again, this workout is entirely optional. If you notice that the inclusion of these workouts diminishes your intensity level on your other workouts, then cut back on your optional cardio time or intensity, or skip it altogether.

You'll perform one of the cardio-based activities listed at a moderate but consistent pace for 30–60 minutes.

TRIPLE THREAT

You'll perform three exercises in a row for 1 minute each. Rest 1 minute, then repeat the triset. Rest 1 minute, then repeat the process with the second triset listed.

Triset 1:
1. Overhead Band Squat
2. Kneeling Dumbbell Overhead Press
3. Speed Skater

Triset 2:
1. Reverse Wood Chopper with Band or Dumbbell (30 seconds per side)
2. Capoeira Sit-Up Plank
3. Cobra-W

OVERHEAD BAND SQUAT: Step on the band and hold the handles in a pronated grip (palms facing forward) with arms extended overhead.

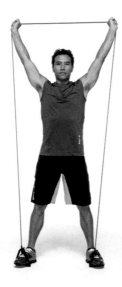
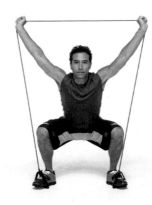

Inhale as you lower yourself down into a squat position, keeping your arms extended above your head until your thighs are parallel to the floor and hips are at knee level.

Exhale as you press through your heels, keeping arms engaged above your head, and return to starting position.

Prefer dumbbells? Start standing with feet shoulder width apart. Hold dumbbells with arms extended above your head, hands shoulder- width apart, arms in line with ears, and palms facing forward. The execution follows the same steps as the band version.

KNEELING DUMBBELL OVERHEAD PRESS: Kneel on the ground on one knee. If using a band, secure the band by kneeling on it and hold each handle in front of your chest at shoulder level with palms facing each other. If using dumbbells, hold the dumbbells in front of your chest at shoulder level with palms facing each other.

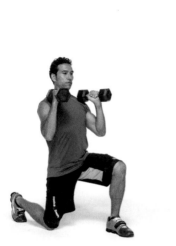
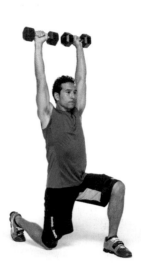

Exhale as you press the dumbbells or band handles directly up toward the ceiling with arms extended above your head in line with your ears, and hands shoulder width apart with palms facing forward. Inhale as you slowly lower the weights back to shoulder level.

SPEED SKATER—LOW: This is a lateral (side-to-side) hopping movement. Stand upright with feet a little wider than shoulders, and with soft knees.

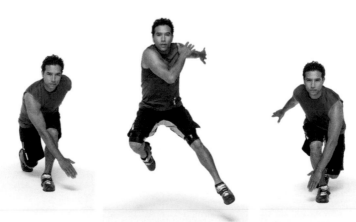

Now, step to the right with your right foot and tuck your left foot behind you, slightly crossed to the outside. Keep your head and upper body facing forward as you bend your knees into a 90/90 position, reaching toward the floor with your left hand and extending your right arm to the side.

Hop to the left with your left foot and tuck your right foot behind your left foot as you reach toward the ground with your right hand.

Reverse the movement, going side to side. Perform this movement as a side-to-side jumping lunge, bending your knees to your level of comfort without trying to touch the ground. Your breathing should be such that you inhale as you land on one side and exhale as you jump to the other.

REVERSE WOOD CHOPPER WITH BAND: Stand upright with your feet wider than shoulder width apart, with toes pointing forward. Step on the band with your left foot. Take the left handle and hold it with your right hand, so that band is stretching from the outside of your left foot to your right hand, with your left hand cupping your right fist.

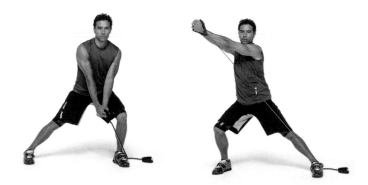

Inhale as you perform a lateral (side) lunge to the left, bending forward slightly, and bringing the band to your left knee. Then, exhale as you stand up and lift the band diagonally across your body to the right side, up to shoulder level. Perform all reps to one side, then switch sides. Be sure to pull in a wide arc with your hands rather than trying to "push" the weight through to the finish.

DUMBBELL VARIATION: Hold one dumbbell above your left shoulder with both hands. Inhale as you perform a lateral (side) lunge to the left, bending forward slightly, and bringing the dumbbell to your left knee. Then, exhale as you stand up and lift the dumbbell diagonally across your body to the right side, up to shoulder level.

CAPOEIRA SIT-UP PLANK: Start lying on your back with knees up, heels on the ground, and hands in front of your chest, chin tucked, looking between your legs, and shoulder blades slightly lifted off the floor.

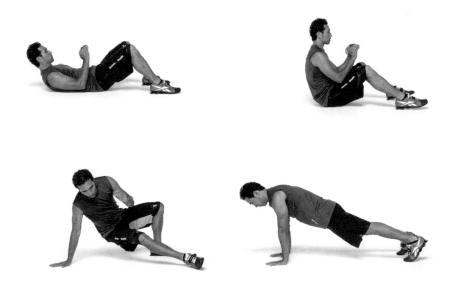

Exhale as you perform a sit-up by engaging your core and lifting your torso off the ground.

Inhale at the top of the sit-up and turn your body to the left to go into a plank position, balancing on your hands and toes.

Exhale as you turn back into the top of the sit-up position. Inhale as you return to the starting position on the ground. Perform the entire movement to the other side.

COBRA-W: Lie facedown on the floor with the laces of your shoes on the floor, and toes pointed, with palms on the floor and hands underneath the shoulders with elbows bent.

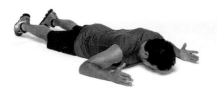 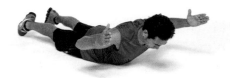

Squeeze your thighs so that your knees lift off the ground. Squeeze your shoulder blades together to lift your elbows slightly. Exhale as you take your hands off the ground, and squeeze your lower, middle, and upper back to lift your upper body off the floor. Perform this version with your arms in a W with elbows bent at 90 degrees, thumbs up to ceiling, and arms raised to ear level.

SCALE IT

Use these versions of the listed exercises to change the degree of difficulty.

OVERHEAD SQUAT WITH BAND OR DUMBBELL: For an easier version, ditch the resistance. To make it harder, press up to a standing position, then perform a single standing shoulder press before descending into a squat again.

KNEELING DUMBBELL OVERHEAD PRESS: To make this exercise easier, decrease the weight or resistance. Or, for a bodyweight option, extend your arms out to the side, palms facing down, to make the letter T with your body, then start fluttering your arms up and down slightly for the full minute. To make this exercise harder, increase the weight or resistance.

SPEED SKATER: To scale this down, perform a "high" speed skater, where you don't go quite as deep on each rep. To increase the difficulty, touch the ground at or near your landing foot on each rep.

REVERSE WOOD CHOPPER WITH BAND: To make this exercise easier, decrease the weight or resistance. Or, for a bodyweight option, ditch the band and replicate the same range of motion, reaching lower toward the floor and higher toward the ceiling on the chop motion for the full minute. To make this exercise harder, increase the weight or resistance.

CAPOEIRA SIT-UP PLANK: For a slightly easier variation, do the plank part of the movement on your knees instead of your toes. A tougher variation calls for a knee strike. When you flip to the plank position on your left side, quickly pull your right knee to your chest as a knee strike. Do the knee strike on the other side during the next rep.

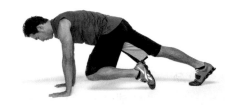

COBRA-W: For a slightly easier version, put your arms in a T position. To make it more advanced, put your arms in a Y.

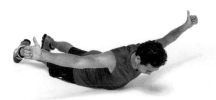
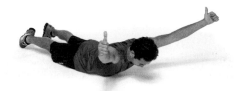

30 HI–30 LO VERSION 3

Perform each exercise listed for 30 seconds and rest for 30 seconds before moving on to the next exercise. It will take 5 minutes to complete one five-exercise circuit. Perform four continuous circuits for a total of 20 minutes.

     1. Burpee
     2. Star Jumps
     3. Push-Up with Release
     4. Mountain Climber
     5. Supported V-Ups

BURPEE: Start in a standing position with legs shoulder width apart.

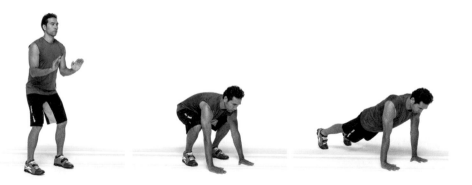

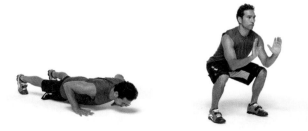

Inhale as you bend down and put your hands on the floor.

Jump your legs behind you to a plank position and do a push-up.

Inhale as you jump to bring your feet back to your hands.

Exhale as you stand up, extending your arms above your head.

STAR JUMPS: This is a combination of a jump squat and a jumping jack. Squat down in the ready position.

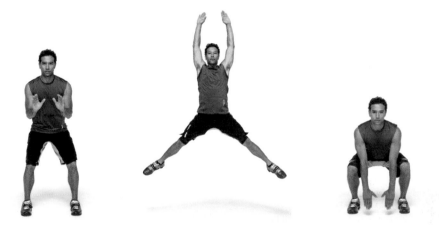

Keep your head and chest pointing forward. Perform a jumping jack with hands and feet in the air, extended out to the sides in a star shape.

Land softly in a squat position. Keep your chest and head forward at all times during this movement. If you were wearing a T-shirt with a number on the front, the number would be visible to someone standing in front of you at all times during this movement.

PUSH-UP WITH RELEASE: Start in a push-up position and lower your body as normal, but pick your hands up off the floor at the bottom of the movement, allowing your chest and hips to make contact with the floor. Replace your hands on the floor underneath your shoulders, then press back to the top.

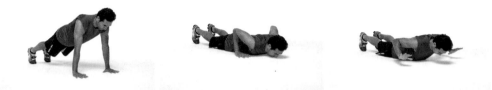

MOUNTAIN CLIMBER: Start in a plank position with your arms fully extended and your hands and toes on the ground. Inhale as you jump your left leg between your hands, keeping your right leg fully extended behind you. Think of bringing your knee to your chest.

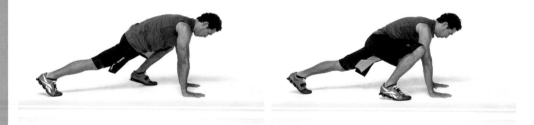

Then, exhale as you jump to reverse your legs. Repeat.

SUPPORTED V-UPS: Sit on the floor with legs extended in front of you. Position your hands on the floor slightly behind your shoulders.

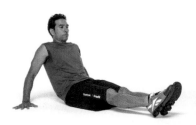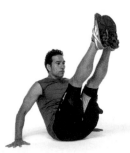

Lift your legs off the ground. Keeping your legs straight, and keeping your hands on the ground, exhale as you hinge your legs toward your torso, and as you move your torso toward your legs.

Inhale as you return legs and torso to the starting position.

SCALE IT

Use these versions of the listed exercises to change the degree of difficulty.

BURPEE: For an easier variation, eliminate the push-up as in a squat-thrust. To increase difficulty, do a sprawl-jump by performing a squat thrust with a sprawl in the plank position, and a jump in the standing position.

STAR JUMPS: A more difficult version would be to either jump your legs higher out to the side or clench your hands in fists when doing the jump. For a less intense version, do a standard jump squat.

PUSH-UP WITH RELEASE: Make any push-up version easier by starting on your knees. To make it tougher, do a plyometric push-up with release, exploding off the floor on each rep and picking your hands and legs up off the floor between reps.

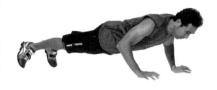

MOUNTAIN CLIMBER: If regular mountain climbers are too difficult to let you sustain a good pace, walk your legs in and out—just slow down a bit. To increase the intensity, perform four mountain climbers in a row. Then, move your hands and feet in a circular motion around to the left. Perform four mountain climbers in this position. Move your hands and feet in a circular motion to the right. Perform four mountain climbers in this position. Repeat.

SUPPORTED V-UPS: An easier variation with similar gains is the abs knee tuck, where you sit on the floor with legs extended in front of you, position your hands on the floor slightly behind your shoulders, lift your legs off the ground with your knees bent at 90 degrees, and exhale as you bring your knees in toward your torso and as you move your head and torso forward. Inhale as you return to the starting position. Repeat for reps. A more difficult version would be to keep your hands off the floor and in front of you as you perform the V-Up. Exhale as you reach for your toes. Inhale as you return to the starting position.

100s

You'll perform two exercises in this workout as a superset, for 10 rounds. One superset consists of 10 reps of each exercise performed back-to-back. Rest 45 seconds before going on to the next superset.

1. Dumbbell Atlas Reverse Lunge (30 seconds each side)
2. Renegade Row with Band or Dumbbell

DUMBBELL ATLAS REVERSE LUNGE: Stand upright, feet shoulder width apart, with dumbbells extended above your head, palms facing forward.

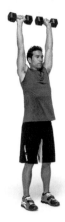
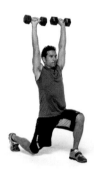
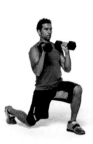

Step your right foot directly back behind you into a reverse lunge, keeping your arms extended straight above your head and in line with your ears.

In this position, at the bottom of the lunge, inhale as you lower the weights to shoulder level in front of your chest with palms facing each other.

Exhale as you press the weights back above your head, palms facing forward. Step your right foot forward to return to the starting position, keeping your arms extended straight above your head. Repeat all reps on the right side, then switch to the left side.

RENEGADE ROW: Perform a push-up with your hands grasping two dumbbells on the floor, your hands facing each other.

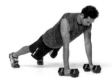
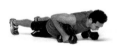
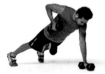

At the top of the push-up, engage your legs and core as you inhale and row the dumbbell up toward your armpit, keeping your elbow alongside your torso.

Exhale as you lower your arm to the ground. Perform the movement again, this time performing a row with the opposite arm. Want a form check? Rest a bottle of water between your shoulder blades. If the bottle rolls off to the left or right, you are over-rotating your hips and/or torso. Strive for total-body control and deep core engagement on this advanced move.

SCALE IT

Use these versions of the listed exercises to change the degree of difficulty.

ATLAS REVERSE LUNGE: For a slightly more tolerable version, skip the overhead press and focus on your lunges. To make it more challenging, bring your rear knee up to waist level on every rep as you press to a full standing position.

RENEGADE ROW: To make this move easier, you can reduce the weight, move your feet farther apart, or try this exercise with just your bodyweight. To make it more difficult, simply increase the weight of the dumbbells or move your feet closer together.

BPS: BODY-PART SPECIFIC

You'll perform two exercises back-to-back, each for a minute. Then you'll rest 30 seconds and move to the next superset. Repeat this for the second superset listed, then move on to the third superset.

Target: Booty
1. Alternating Side Lunges
2. 1-Leg Booty Bridge-V on Heels (30 seconds per side)

Target: Chest
1. Chest Fly with Band or Chest Fly Booty Bridge
2. 1-Leg Push-Up with Band

Target: Abs

    1. Capoeira Push Kick Sit-Up (*Bênção* Sit-Up)

    2. Forearm Plank Jack

ALTERNATING SIDE LUNGES: Stand upright with feet shoulder width apart and with arms at your sides.

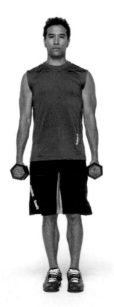
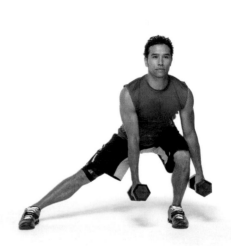

Keep your left leg straight as you inhale and step out to the right side in a wide step with your right leg. Bend your leg as you lunge down deeply, touching the floor with both hands on either side of your right foot, while keeping your chest up and eyes on the horizon.

Exhale as you return to the starting position. Alternate sides.

20-DAY FITNESS PLAN: BLUE

1-LEG BOOTY BRIDGE-V ON HEELS: Start lying on your back with your arms along your sides, palms up, and your left knee up with left foot on the floor close to your hips with your toes up. Your right leg is extended straight along the floor with toes pointing up.

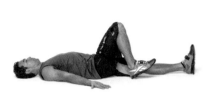 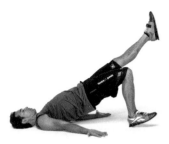

Engage your core as you exhale and press through your left heel to lift your hips to knee level while raising your right leg until your thighs are parallel, with your right leg extended.

Inhale as you lower your body back to the starting position. Take care not to twist the raised leg outward—always picture a glass of water being balanced on your belt buckle.

CHEST FLY WITH BAND: Begin in a lunge position with left leg forward and right leg behind you. Hold the handles of the exercise band with your arms extended to each side, stepping on the band with your right leg. Face your palms forward.

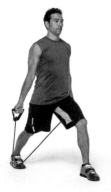 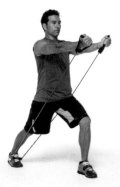

Exhale as you slowly move your arms forward in a semicircle, stopping just before your palms touch in front of you at your bust. Picture yourself driving your elbows and palms toward each other at the top of the movement.

Inhale as you let your arms retrace the semicircle backward to the starting position.

DUMBBELL CHEST FLY BOOTY BRIDGE: Position yourself in a stable, booty bridge position holding a pair of dumbbells out at your sides with your arms in a T and a slight bend in your elbows.

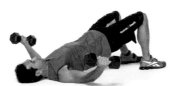 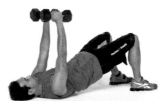

Exhale as you move the dumbbells up in a wide arc until they touch, then inhale as you slowly return them to the start position.

1-LEG PUSH-UP WITH BAND: Perform the push-up while keeping one leg raised a few inches off the ground and fully extended. Switch legs for the next rep.

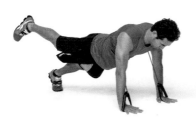 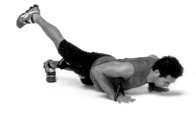

CAPOEIRA PUSH KICK SIT-UP (*BÊNÇÃO* SIT-UP): Inhale as you perform the sit-up while drawing your left knee into your chest with your left foot flexed and your hands up.

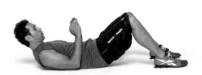 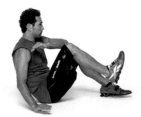

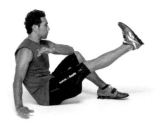

Exhale as you push your left leg out in front of you, leading with your heel, and sweep your right arm across your face with elbow bent at 90 degrees and your left arm extended to the left side.

Inhale as you bring your knee back to your chest. Exhale as you return to starting position and repeat on the other side.

FOREARM PLANK JACK: Perform a forearm plank. Exhale as you jump your feet out wider than your shoulders.

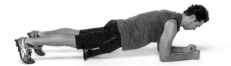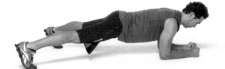

Inhale as you jump your feet back to the starting position. Repeat.

SCALE IT

Use these versions of the listed exercises to change the degree of difficulty.

ALTERNATING SIDE LUNGES: To make this easier, bend your knees less during the lunge. To increase the demand, do all reps on one side for 30 straight seconds, then switch.

SINGLE-LEG BOOTY BRIDGE-V ON HEELS: To make it slightly easier, you can alternate legs. To increase the difficulty, you can add a little swing. When your leg is raised, swing the leg out to the side without turning your hips. Return to the starting position.

CHEST FLY WITH BAND OR CHEST FLY BOOTY BRIDGE WITH DUMBBELLS: If the weighted version is too challenging, scale down by simply performing a wide push-up from the knees. To make it more advanced, with the band, step on the band with back leg, arms at sides, palms facing forward. Bring arms forward to chest level, palms facing in. Add a short pulse rep after you bring palms together. To increase the demand with dumbbells, lie on your back with hips bridged up off floor on your heels, arms out to the side with slight bend in elbow, palms facing up. When arms are apart at bottom, add a short pulse rep before lifting arms in a wide arc to top.

1-LEG PUSH-UP WITH BAND: To make this easier, just perform a regular push-up. To spice up this move and really hit your core, booty, and hips, perform a leg swing with one leg out to the side as you inhale and lower yourself into the push-up. Exhale as you press up and pull your leg back into the starting position. The key on the leg swing is to first engage your stationary leg and core before swinging your leg out.

CAPOEIRA PUSH KICK SIT-UP (*BÊNÇÃO* SIT-UP): The capoeira knee tuck sit-up is an adequate modifier if this version is too tough. Lie on your back with your fists at your chest. Bend your knees and place your feet on the floor. Inhale as you sit up, drawing your left knee into your chest, keeping your foot flexed and hands up. Exhale as you return to the starting position. Repeat on your right side. To go with a more advanced move, perform the push kick sit-up as described above, but as you lower yourself to the ground, do the "Shake & Bake" by twisting your torso back and forth.

FOREARM PLANK JACK: You can simplify this advanced move a bit by performing a regular plank, alternating between being on your knees and being on your toes for time. For a slightly different emphasis, perform a forearm single-leg plank variation. Lift one leg off the ground and tap your toe to the ground. Repeat on the other side. Switch sides and continue the toe-tap motion throughout the movement.

20-DAY FITNESS Q&A

Answers to a few of the questions you're bound to be asking in the next 20 days.

Q: What if I have to miss a workout?

A: If you can't get your workout in on a particular day, get creative! Do you have a staircase at work? If you do, run up and down the stairs for 10 minutes two times during the day. Park farther away than you need to, or get off the bus a stop or two early and power-walk the rest of the way. Work movement into your day any way that you can, and then get back on your workout schedule tomorrow, no questions asked.

Q: What if working out in the morning makes me feel tired?

A: The United States is one of the only places in the world where people don't have a cultural habit of napping even though it's one of the best things we can do for our health. How many times have you looked to a vending machine for a mid-afternoon pick-me-up? Trust me—a nap or a brisk walk is much better for you and will do much more for your overall health.

If your schedule permits it, try closing your eyes for 20 minutes when you're most tired in the afternoon. Even if you don't fall deeply asleep, you'll be more rested and alert when you rise.

Q: **What if I can't do an exercise the way you're teaching it, owing to pain or physical limitations?**

A: Don't worry! As I said, no two bodies are alike. You can always modify an exercise if doing it the way it's pictured here leads to pain or too much soreness, or if it just doesn't fit your body. For example, if you experience wrist pain in the plank position, try doing a plank on your forearms instead. If just being in that position is uncomfortable, do the movement against a sofa, a staircase, or a wall. If an exercise calls for an explosive movement (a jump, for example), you can always keep one foot on the ground to modify the movement. It won't be quite as strenuous an exercise, but it will still give you great benefits. My test groups for the *20-Minute Body* program included individuals who had to use these modifications all the time, and they still came away with great results. I offer easier—as well as more advanced—modifications for every exercise in this book so you can choose the level of comfort that suits you best. If you find that you are struggling after only a few reps, go ahead and modify with the easier options provided.

Be creative with your workouts and always remember that you should never perform an exercise that causes acute pain. Muscle soreness is okay—even desirable—but acute pain is not. Be honest with yourself about injuries if you expect to get through any workout program. Otherwise, things could get much worse and before you know it, you could suffer a catastrophic injury. Modify any movement that you need to modify in order to continue training and seeing results.

Q: **What if my weight loss hits a plateau?**

A: Weight loss can stall for a number of reasons. Make sure that you're eating enough (so you don't feel excessively hungry), and that you're eating the most nutritious foods. If you can't seem to shake the extra weight, try adding a cardio-air workout in place of your dedicated rest day of each week. Also, be aware of how much sodium is in the food you are consuming: if you eat a high-sodium meal the night before you check your weight, you could easily be holding on to a couple of pounds of excess water weight. Also, acute inflammation from the new workout can cause you to show a few pounds heavier. If you've been at it a few weeks, you may have made a swap in the right direction, adding two pounds of muscle and losing a pound of fat, showing a net gain of a pound.

Remember: the scale is not your best indicator of progress. Be sure to track your measurements and the fit of your clothes *as well as* your scale weight, since your body composition is likely to change.

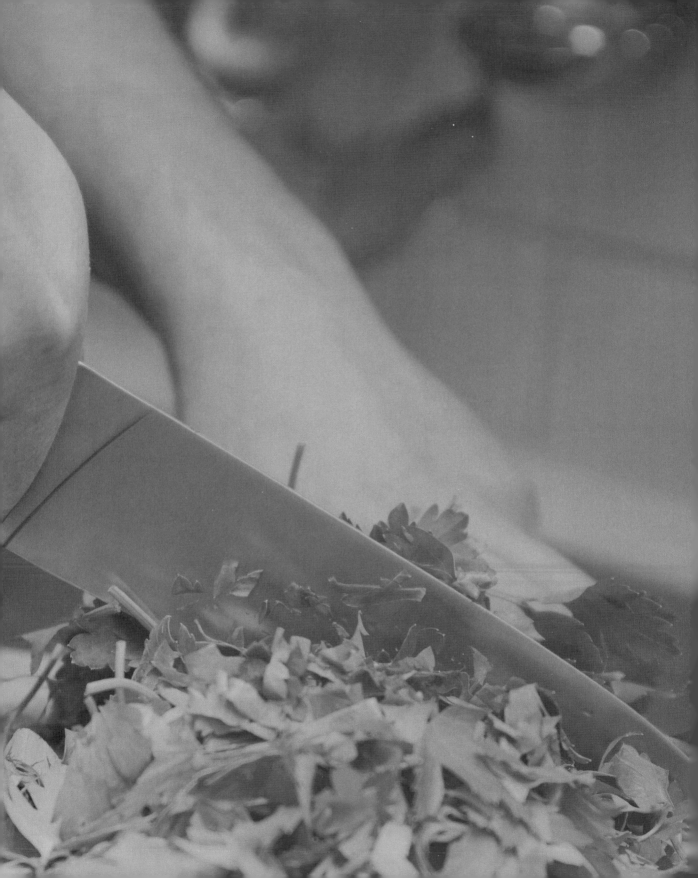

TWELVE

The 20-Day Meal Plan

REMEMBER... EATING LEAN, CLEAN, AND GREEN is what supports your quest to develop metabolic muscle. You break it down in the workouts —this is what builds it up! All the workouts that you'll be doing are the stimulus for change, but the real results are had in the kitchen.

But you also don't want to break the bank doing it. These meal plans are designed to allow for the occasional date with leftovers. Many dishes reheat well and this will be a huge asset to you when it comes to condensing your meal prep times. Most of the recipes are designed to make four servings, but you'll find in many cases that you are cooking more than what's needed. This is called batch cooking and it's a nutritional time-saver that many pro athletes, models, and busy professionals use to keep on track.

Let's get cooking!

20-DAY MEAL PLAN: YELLOW

At this level, you'll get seven days' worth of recipes that you can repeat as you like—or you can use the meal plan to schedule your cooking. I'm also recommending a Sunday start—people like to start "diets" on a Monday, but that usually leads them to gorge on Sunday. This ensures that you're starting your week feeling good. No more Monday food hangovers! But that's just my suggestion. You should start on the day that is most convenient for you.

Walk yourself through the calendar so you can see that I meant it when I said you'd be eating many of the same tasty foods that you're already feeding your family! These just have a little extra "health" on the side—energy-packed ingredients, slow-digesting carbs, and tons of vitamins.

SHOPPING LIST: YELLOW

It's all about the basics. Lean proteins, fresh fruits and vegetables, foods close to their natural state. In other words, less lab, more lean! Here is the shopping list for your first 20 days. It's important to note that the lists and recipes were created to serve four; so if you are cooking only for yourself, or for two, be sure to scale down as needed.

WEEK 1

PRODUCE

1 pound romaine lettuce
2 pounds baby spinach
Two 10-ounce bunches kale
3 heads broccoli
3 bags carrots
3 red bell peppers
1 green bell pepper
1 jalapeño pepper
5 avocados
2 cucumbers
3 large zucchini

1½ pounds green beans
2 bunches celery
One 5-ounce package
    mushrooms
1 medium yellow onion
3 red onions
2 heads garlic
8 medium sweet potatoes
    or yams
1 tomato
2 bunches fresh cilantro

1 bunch fresh parsley

1 bunch fresh mint

I head napa or savoy
    cabbage

1 bunch bananas

1 pear

5 apples

4 limes

2 lemons

2 small oranges

2 containers of berries
    (blueberries, raspberries,
    or strawberries)

DAIRY

4 dozen eggs

One 8-ounce container
    freshly grated Parmesan
    cheese

One 8-ounce bag grated
    cheddar cheese

One 8-ounce bag grated
    mozzarella cheese

1 gallon organic skim milk

35 ounces plain, 2% Greek
    yogurt

One 8-ounce container
    sour cream

½ pound feta cheese

The progression of these meal plans is designed to lead you toward better choices. Cow's milk, as previously discussed, is not an ideal choice, but many people depend on it as a staple of their nutrition. Cow's milk and products made from it are allowed in this phase—choose organic, if possible—but will be replaced gradually with alternatives such as coconut milk later on.

MEAT

1 pound ground turkey

1 pound boneless, skinless
    chicken breasts

1 pound 90–93% lean
    ground beef

1 pound salmon fillets

1 pound cod fillets

1 pound medium peeled,
    deveined shrimp (about
    22)

FROZEN

12 ounces frozen sweet
    potato fries

2 pounds frozen whole
    wheat pizza dough

OILS, CONDIMENTS, SPICES

One 5-ounce can cooking
    spray

One 25-ounce bottle olive oil

One 14-ounce jar coconut
    oil

One 26-ounce container
    sea salt

One 2-ounce container
    black pepper

One 2-ounce jar mild chili powder

One 2-ounce jar dried herbs, such as thyme

One 2-ounce jar ground cumin

One 2-ounce jar ground cinnamon

One 2-ounce jar garlic powder

One 2-ounce bottle vanilla extract

One 2-ounce bottle rum extract

One 6-ounce can Old Bay Seasoning

One 10-ounce bottle white or balsamic vinegar

One 8-ounce jar mustard

One 15-ounce jar olive oil– based mayonnaise

One 15-ounce jar salsa

One 10-ounce bottle low sodium soy sauce

One 5-ounce bottle hot sauce

One 8-ounce container unsweetened cocoa powder

One 16-ounce jar almond or peanut butter

One 12-ounce container whey protein powder

One 8-ounce bottle real maple syrup

One package bamboo skewers

A blend of several herbs and spices, Old Bay still contains some salt. Opt for the lower-sodium version if available. If you can't find it, Konriko brand seasoning salt—Chipotle or Jalapeño—is also a good choice.

GRAINS AND DRY GROCERIES

1 small bag whole wheat bread crumbs

2 small whole wheat pitas

4 whole wheat 100-calorie sandwich flats

12 corn taco shells or small corn tortillas

Eight 6-inch whole wheat flour tortillas

8 slices whole-grain or whole wheat bread

One 42-ounce container old-fashioned oats

One 16-ounce bag shredded unsweetened flaked coconut

One 8-ounce box whole wheat or whole-grain pasta, such as mini penne or spirals

One 8-ounce box whole wheat or whole-grain spaghetti

One 14-ounce box instant brown rice

One 16-ounce bag chia seeds

One 16-ounce bag ground flaxseed

One 12-ounce box raisins

One 1-pound box brown sugar or 1 container granulated Stevia

One 8-ounce bag walnuts

CANNED AND JARRED GOODS

One 15-ounce can pumpkin

One 5-ounce can chipotle peppers in adobe sauce

Two 5-ounce cans tomato paste

Two 15-ounce cans diced tomatoes

Two 15-ounce cans low-sodium beans, any variety

One 15-ounce can chickpeas

One 15-ounce can black beans

One 10-ounce container pitted olives, such as kalamata

Two 32-ounce containers low-sodium chicken or vegetable broth

WEEK 2

PRODUCE

Two 10-ounce bunches kale

2 pounds baby spinach

1 pound romaine lettuce

2 bags carrots

2 bunches celery

4 red onions

2 heads garlic

3 tomatoes

8 Hass avocados

2 green bell peppers

2 red bell peppers

2 jalapeño peppers

1 zucchini

1 cucumber

1 bunch asparagus

1 head napa or savoy cabbage

Three 5-ounce packages mushrooms, such as button or cremini

1 pound green beans

2 heads broccoli

1 bunch fresh mint

1 bunch fresh parsley

1 bunch cilantro

1 bunch scallions

10 sweet potatoes or yams (about 6 pounds)

3 lemons

6 limes

1 pear

4 apples

3 pints fresh berries, such as raspberries, black-berries, or blueberries

MEAT

1 pound cubed beef stew meat

1 pound ground turkey

3 pounds boneless, skinless chicken breasts (about 3 large or 4 small)

2 pounds 90–93% lean ground beef

1 pound cod fillets

1 pound salmon fillets, skin on

DAIRY

½ gallon organic skim milk

½ gallon plain unsweetened coconut milk

2 dozen eggs

One 5-ounce container crumbled feta

One 32-ounce container plain, 2% Greek yogurt

8 ounces shredded cheddar cheese

8 ounces shredded mozzarella cheese

FROZEN

1 pound frozen whole wheat pizza dough

OILS, CONDIMENTS, SPICES

One 15-ounce jar salsa

One 2-ounce bottle cardamom

One 2-ounce bottle oregano

One 2-ounce bottle dried parsley

One 2-ounce bottle onion powder

One 2-ounce bottle nutmeg

One 2-ounce bottle ginger

One 2-ounce bottle cayenne pepper

GRAINS AND DRY GROCERIES

One 26-ounce container whole-grain pancake mix

4 small whole wheat buns (about 100 calories apiece)

4 small (6-inch) whole wheat pitas

4 whole wheat 100-calorie sandwich flats

Four 9-inch whole wheat wraps (around 160 calories apiece)

One 3-ounce bag sweet potato chips

Eight 6-inch whole wheat flour tortillas

8 slices whole-grain or whole wheat bread

One 14-ounce box instant brown rice

One 12-ounce bag bittersweet chocolate chips

One 10-ounce bag walnuts

One 4-ounce bar 70% cocoa

JARRED AND CANNED GOODS

One 24-ounce jar low-sodium marinara sauce

One 12-ounce jar honey

One 16-ounce jar peanut butter

Two 15-ounce cans diced tomatoes

Two 32-ounce containers low-sodium chicken broth

Two 15-ounce cans low-sodium beans

Two 15-ounce cans chickpeas

Two 15-ounce cans black beans

Two 5-ounce cans tomato paste

One 10-ounce jar black olives

WEEK 3

PRODUCE

2 pounds green beans

One 10-ounce bunch kale

1 head savory or napa cabbage

2 pounds baby spinach

3 pounds asparagus

1 zucchini

1 head romaine or butter lettuce

1 head broccoli

Three 5-ounce containers mushrooms

2 red bell peppers

1 green bell pepper

1 jalapeño pepper

1 head garlic

1 small gingerroot

2 large sweet potatoes

3 Hass avocados

4 red onions

1 bunch basil or parsley

1 bag celery

1 tomato

1 bunch fresh mint

1 bunch fresh parsley

1 bunch fresh cilantro

1 pear

2 bananas

3 limes

1 pound fresh berries, such as raspberries, blueberries, or blackberries

2 lemons

4 apples

DAIRY

3 dozen eggs

One 8-ounce container grated Parmesan cheese

Two 15-ounce containers part-skim ricotta cheese

1 pound grated part-skim mozzarella cheese

½ gallon organic skim milk

One 32-ounce container plain 2% Greek yogurt

One 8-ounce package nitrate-free bacon

8 ounces shredded part-skim mozzarella cheese

8 ounces shredded cheddar cheese

4 ounces feta cheese

MEAT, POULTRY, AND FISH

3 pounds 90–93% lean ground beef

2 pounds boneless, skinless chicken breasts

2 pounds cod fillets

1 pound salmon

1 pound shrimp, shelled and deveined

FROZEN

1 pound frozen whole wheat pizza dough

2 pounds frozen blueberries or raspberries

GRAINS AND DRY GROCERIES

2 packages whole wheat flour tortillas

1 loaf whole-grain or whole wheat bread

Two 1-pound boxes whole wheat spaghetti

One 12-ounce box whole wheat lasagna noodles

1 package (6-inch) whole wheat pitas

One 12-ounce container vanilla protein powder

One 12-ounce container chocolate protein powder

One 14-ounce box instant brown rice

OILS, CONDIMENTS, SPICES

One 25-ounce bottle olive oil

1 12-ounce jar cocktail sauce

JARRED AND CANNED GOODS

Two 24-ounce jars low sodium marinara sauce

Two 15-ounce cans chickpeas

One 15-ounce container low-sodium chicken or vegetable broth

One 5-ounce container almonds

One 15-ounce can black beans

Two 5-ounce cans tomato paste

20-DAY MEAL PLAN: YELLOW

DAY 1

BREAKFAST

Frittata

Chef's Note: Save leftovers to make Day 3's breakfast.

LUNCH

Empanada

Chef's Note: Defrost extra pizza dough to make empanadas for Day 3's lunch.

SNACK

Chipotle or Pesto Deviled Eggs

DINNER

Turkey Tacos

Chef's Notes: Get a head start on the rest of the week by cooking sweet potatoes in the slow cooker. Make a big batch of the base for the turkey tacos (same as turkey chili) to use throughout the week.

DESSERT

Baked Apples

Chef's Note: Yes, dessert happens here. Cook enough to use throughout the week!

DAY 2

BREAKFAST

Beta Blaster Smoothie

LUNCH

Burrito

Chef's Note: This is made with leftover turkey meat from tacos on Day 1.

SNACK

Chocolate Peanut Butter Banana
Shake

DINNER

Minestrone

Chef's Notes: This is leftover from
Day 1 prep. Today, defrost pizza
dough for calzone.

DAY 3

BREAKFAST

Frittata

Chef's Note: No prep this morning!
This is leftover from Day 1. Just
take it out of the fridge, reheat, and
enjoy!

LUNCH

Calzone or Empanada

SNACK

Peanut Satay Dip

Chef's Note: Make double the dip to
use with dinner on Day 4.

DINNER

Orange Thyme Salmon or
Honey Glazed Salmon

DESSERT

Frozen Yogurt Pops

DAY 4

BREAKFAST

Baked Apple Parfait

Chef's Note: Use leftover slow-
cooker apples if you have them.

LUNCH

Bunless Salmon Burgers

Chef's Note: Use leftover salmon from last night's dinner for this lunch.

SNACK

Kale Chips or Truffles

DINNER

Chicken Peanut Satay

Chef's Note: You can use leftover dip from snack on Day 3.

DAY 5

BREAKFAST

Cinnamon Nut Breakfast Cereal

LUNCH

Sloppy Joes

Chef's Note: You can use leftover turkey taco meat.

SNACK

Guacamole with 1 cup veggies

DINNER

Coconut Shrimp

DAY 6

BREAKFAST

Minty Lean and Green Shake

LUNCH

Lemon Pepper Chicken Veggie Bowl

Chef's Note: You can cook fresh if you want or, to cut time, you can use leftover chicken skewer meat from Day 4.

SNACK
Leftover Trail Mix or Kale Chips

DINNER
Tilapia Tacos

DAY 7

BREAKFAST
French Toast

LUNCH
Italian Meat Loaf

SNACK
Chipotle or Pesto Deviled Eggs

DINNER
Sweet Potato Stuffer

DESSERT
Bananas Foster Parfait

DAY 8

BREAKFAST
Frittata

Chef's Note: Save leftovers to make Day 10's breakfast.

LUNCH
Empanada

Chef's Note: Defrost extra pizza dough to make empanadas for Day 10's lunch.

SNACK
Chipotle or Pesto Deviled Eggs

DINNER

Turkey Tacos

Chef's Notes: Get a head start on the rest of the week by cooking sweet potatoes in the slow cooker. Make a big batch of the base for the turkey tacos (same as turkey chili) to use throughout the week.

DESSERT

Baked Apples

Chef's Note: Cook enough to use throughout the week!

DAY 9

BREAKFAST

Beta Blaster Smoothie

LUNCH

Burrito

Chef's Note: This is made with leftover turkey meat from tacos on Day 8.

SNACK

Chocolate Peanut Butter Banana Shake

DINNER

Minestrone

Chef's Notes: This is leftover from Day 8 prep. Today, defrost pizza dough for calzone.

DAY 10

BREAKFAST

Frittata

Chef's Note: No prep this morning! This is leftover from Day 1. Just take it out of the fridge, reheat, and enjoy!

LUNCH

Calzone or Empanada

SNACK

Peanut Satay Dip

Chef's Note: Make double the dip to use with dinner on Day 11.

DINNER

Orange Thyme Salmon or Honey Glazed Salmon

DESSERT

Frozen Yogurt Pops

DAY 11

BREAKFAST

Baked Apple Parfait

Chef's Note: Use leftover baked apples if you have them.

LUNCH

Bunless Salmon Burgers

Chef's Note: Use leftover salmon from last night's dinner for this lunch.

SNACK

Kale Chips or Truffles

DINNER

Chicken Peanut Satay

Chef's Note: You can use leftover dip from snack on Day 10.

DAY 12

BREAKFAST

Cinnamon Nut Breakfast Cereal

LUNCH

Sloppy Joes

Chef's Note: You can use leftover turkey taco meat.

SNACK

Guacamole with 1 cup veggies

DINNER

Coconut Shrimp

DAY 13

BREAKFAST

Minty Lean and Green Shake

LUNCH

Lemon Pepper Chicken Veggie Bowl

Chef's Note: You can cook fresh if you want or, to cut time, you can use leftover chicken skewer meat from Day 11.

SNACK

Leftover Trail Mix or Kale Chips

DINNER

Cod Tacos

DAY 14

BREAKFAST

French Toast

LUNCH

Italian Meat Loaf

SNACK

Chipotle or Pesto Deviled Eggs

DINNER

Sweet Potato Stuffer

DESSERT

Bananas Foster Parfait

DAY 15

BREAKFAST

Frittata

Chef's Note: Save leftovers to make Day 17's breakfast.

LUNCH

Empanada

Chef's Note: Defrost extra pizza dough to make empanadas for Day 17's lunch.

SNACK

Chipotle or Pesto Deviled Eggs

DINNER

Turkey Tacos

Chef's Notes: Get a head start on the rest of the week by cooking sweet potatoes in the slow cooker. Make a big batch of the base for the turkey tacos (same as turkey chili) to use throughout the week.

DESSERT

Baked Apples

Chef's Note: Cook enough to use throughout the week!

DAY 16

BREAKFAST

Beta Blaster Smoothie

LUNCH

Burrito

Chef's Note: This is made with leftover turkey meat from tacos on Day 15.

SNACK

Chocolate Peanut Butter Banana Shake

DINNER

Minestrone

Chef's Notes: This is leftover from Day 15 prep. Today, defrost pizza dough for calzone.

DAY 17

BREAKFAST

Frittata

Chef's Note: No prep this morning! This is leftover from Day 15. Just take it out of the fridge, reheat, and enjoy!

LUNCH

Calzone or Empanada

SNACK

Peanut Satay Dip

Chef's Note: Make double the dip to use with dinner on Day 18.

DINNER

Orange Thyme Salmon or Honey Glazed Salmon

DESSERT

Berry Delicious Frozen Yogurt Pops

DAY 18

BREAKFAST

Baked Apple Parfait

Chef's Note: Use leftover baked apples if you have them.

LUNCH

Bunless Salmon Burgers

Chef's Note: Use leftover salmon from last night's dinner for this lunch.

SNACK

Kale Chips or Truffles

DINNER

Chicken Peanut Satay

Chef's Note: You can use leftover dip from snack on Day 17.

DAY 19

BREAKFAST

Cinnamon Nut Breakfast Cereal

LUNCH

Sloppy Joes

Chef's Note: You can use leftover turkey taco meat.

SNACK

Guacamole with 1 cup veggies

DINNER

Coconut Shrimp

DAY 20

BREAKFAST

Minty Lean and Green Shake

LUNCH

Lemon Pepper Chicken Veggie
Bowl

Chef's Note: You can cook fresh if
you want or, to cut time, you can
use leftover chicken skewer meat
from Day 18.

SNACK

Leftover Trail Mix or Kale Chips

DINNER

Cod Tacos

20-DAY RECIPES: YELLOW

You may remember that I said I was as much a novice in the kitchen as anyone else. I could always manage to get by, but when it came to seasoning things or organizing the meal prep, I was anything but an expert. But I soon realized that you don't need to have the culinary savvy of Chef Rocco to cook healthy meals. These recipes on the yellow level are super easy for anyone to follow. If I can make 'em, you can make 'em!

I've grouped these recipes into breakfasts, snacks, lunches, dinners and—*wait for it*—desserts, to serve as a quick guide for finding the directions you need.

BREAKFASTS

VEGGIE FRITTATA

This no-brainer frittata recipe is ideal for newbie egg cooks, since it bakes in the oven, no flipping required. It also reheats beautifully, so it is a great breakfast or snack to take on the road. Reheat in a microwave on low for 20 seconds or in a toaster oven for 10 minutes at 400°F.

Serves 4

1 tablespoon olive oil
1 red bell pepper, seeded and thinly sliced
1 large zucchini, diced
½ medium onion, diced
4 garlic cloves, unpeeled
¼ cup chopped fresh parsley and cilantro
⅛ teaspoon salt
6 eggs
⅓ cup finely shredded Parmesan cheese
¼ teaspoon chili powder
Cooking spray
2 small whole wheat pitas, cut in half, toasted

Preheat the oven to 400°F. Place a large skillet over medium heat. Add the olive oil along with the bell pepper, zucchini, onion, garlic, parsley, and cilantro. Sprinkle with salt. Cook 3 to 4 minutes, stirring occasionally, until the vegetables start to soften. Transfer the veggies to a plate.

Scramble the eggs with the Parmesan cheese and the chili powder. Carefully coat the skillet with the cooking spray. Add the egg mixture and cook 2 to 3 minutes, pulling the edges of the cooked egg once or twice into the center of the pan.

Top with the cooked veggies and transfer to the oven. Cook 8 to 10 minutes, until the egg is cooked through. Remove from oven and rest 5 minutes before slicing into 4 pie-shaped wedges and serving with the pitas.

Nutritional Stats Per serving (serving size: 7 ounces plus ½ small pita) 282 calories, 17 g protein, 5 g sugars, 25 g carbohydrates, 14 g fat (4 g saturated), 284 mg cholesterol, 4 g fiber, 473 mg sodium

BETA BLASTER

Get great skin with this low-calorie breakfast—it's high in beta-carotene from everyday foods like carrots and pumpkin. New research says that getting plenty of foods rich in beta-carotene may help turn the tide when it comes to diseases like diabetes.

Serves 2

    1 cup organic skim milk
    ½ cup plain, 2% Greek yogurt
    4 ice cubes
    1 apple, cored, skin on
    2 carrots, peeled
    ¼ cup canned pumpkin
    2 tablespoons ground flaxseed
    2 tablespoons almond butter or peanut butter
    1 tablespoon brown sugar
    1 teaspoon cinnamon

Place all ingredients in a blender and blend until smooth. Serve immediately.

Chef's Note: Refer to page 115 for blenders. The Ninja blender would be good for this—or the Magic Bullet, which is ideal for those with little or no storage space.

Nutritional Stats Per serving (serving size: 1½ cups) 318 calories, 15 g protein, 27 g sugars, 40 g carbohydrates, 13 g fat (2 g saturated), 6 mg cholesterol, 9 g fiber, 117 mg sodium

BAKED APPLE BREAKFAST PARFAIT

Need more time for your workout? Make your leftovers work for you and use leftover baked apples. You can also double the recipe for baked apples, cool them, and freeze them for impromptu parfaits.

Serves 4

8 baked apple halves
2 cups plain, 2% Greek yogurt
2 teaspoons brown sugar

Cut each of the baked apple halves into four even strips. Place the yogurt in a small bowl and add the brown sugar. Stir well.

Layer ¼ cup of the yogurt mixture into four glasses, top each layer with two slices of the apple, repeat with remaining yogurt and apple slices, and serve.

Nutritional Stats Per serving (serving size: 1 parfait) 317 calories, 12 g protein, 34 g sugars, 41 g carbohydrates, 14 g fat (3 g saturated), 8 mg cholesterol, 5 g fiber, 38 mg sodium

CINNAMON NUT BREAKFAST CEREAL

Oats are touted for their ability to rope in LDL, or "bad" cholesterol, because they are rich in soluble fiber that grabs onto free-floating cholesterol and whisks it out of your system. Berries are oats' best buds, because they add sweet taste and another huge hit of fiber, which can also slow the uptake of nutrients, helping to prevent spikes in blood sugar for a leaner body.

Serves 4

2 cup old-fashioned oats
5 cups water
4 scoops protein powder (1⅓ cups)
1 tablespoon brown sugar

1 teaspoon cinnamon
¼ cup chopped nuts, such as walnuts or almonds
1 cup fresh berries, such as raspberries or blueberries

Place the oats, protein powder, brown sugar, and cinnamon in a medium saucepan. Add 5 cups of water and bring to a simmer over medium-low heat. Cook 4 to 5 minutes, stirring often, until the oats are tender. Top with nuts and berries. Serve immediately.

Nutritional Stats Per serving (serving size: 2 cups) 324 calories, 25 g protein, 7 g sugars, 40 g carbohydrates, 10 g fat (2 g saturated), 0 mg cholesterol, 10 g fiber, 81 mg sodium

Chef's Note: Ground cardamom is a peppery spice, used in international baking, that has a hint of mint. For a flavor twist try adding a pinch of ground cardamom or freshly grated nutmeg to your hot cereal.

MINTY LEAN AND GREEN SHAKE

This frothy, light green shake calls for mint to sweeten the vegetal flavor of kale, king of the superfoods. Just 1 cup of kale provides a host of vital nutrients like 100 percent of your vitamin C needs, plus other nutrients to fuel your busy day—like vitamin A, iron, and folate to name just a few. Juicy pear provides plenty of fiber along with sweet fruit flavor.

Serves 2

1 cup kale
2 stalks celery
1 pear, seeded
2 scoops protein powder (about ⅔ cup)
2 cups skim milk
2 tablespoons fresh mint
1 tablespoon brown sugar
8 ice cubes

Place all the ingredients in a blender and blend until very smooth. Serve immediately.

Nutritional Stats Per serving (serving size: 1½ cups) 272 calories, 28 g protein, 28 g sugars, 40 g carbohydrates, 2 g fat (1 g saturated), 5 mg cholesterol, 7 g fiber, 232 mg sodium

FRENCH TOAST

French toast is a decadent breakfast, but it doesn't mean you can't bump up the nutrition. Adding ground flaxseed to the mix makes French toast a surprising way to get a good dose of fiber.

Serves 4

1 cup organic skim milk
2 eggs
2 tablespoons ground flaxseed
1 tablespoon brown sugar
1 teaspoon vanilla extract
¼ teaspoon ground cinnamon
8 slices whole-grain or whole wheat bread
Cooking spray
1 cup fresh berries, such as raspberries or blueberries
¼ cup real maple syrup

Place the milk, eggs, flaxseed, sugar, vanilla, and cinnamon in a large, shallow bowl and whisk well. Using the tines of a fork, poke the bread several times to allow better absorption of the liquid.

Coat a large skillet with cooking spray and place it over medium heat. Dip four of the bread slices into the egg mixture and transfer to skillet. Cook 2 to 3 minutes per side until golden, then turn. Cook 2 to 3 minutes more until a crisp crust has formed. Transfer to a plate and repeat with cooking spray and remaining bread. Top with berries and drizzle with syrup. Serve immediately.

Nutritional Stats Per serving (serving size: 2 slices French toast, ¼ cup berries, plus 1 tablespoon syrup): 354 calories, 14 g protein, 27 g sugars, 64 g carbohydrates, 4 g fat (1 g saturated), 94 mg cholesterol, 9 g fiber, 446 mg sodium

SNACKS

CHIPOTLE OR PESTO DEVILED EGGS

If you're feeling blue during the winter months, eggs are a great superfood to include in your diet, as long as you eat the yolk, too! The yolk is rich in two vital mood-lifting nutrients: choline, a major brain food that also fights accumulations of fat in your liver; and vitamin D, the sunshine vitamin.

Serves 4

8 eggs
¼ cup olive oil–based mayonnaise
2 tablespoons chipotle peppers in adobo sauce, chopped, or pesto recipe (page 265 or 342)

Place the eggs in a saucepan. Fill with cold water. Place over high heat and bring to a boil. Cover and rest off the heat for 15 minutes. Drain and rinse under cold water to peel.

Cut the eggs in half lengthwise and scoop out the yolks. Transfer the yolks to a medium bowl along with the mayonnaise and the chipotle or pesto. Mix well with a fork, breaking up the yolk with a fork as you mix.

Transfer the yolk mixture back into the egg halves and serve immediately or transfer to an airtight container and store refrigerated for up to 3 days.

Nutritional Stats Per serving (serving size: 2 deviled eggs) 200 calories, 13 g protein, 0 g sugars, 2 g carbohydrates, 15 g fat (4 g saturated), 377 mg cholesterol, 0 g fiber, 297 mg sodium

CHOCOLATE PEANUT BUTTER BANANA SHAKE

Chocolate, peanut butter, and bananas are three ingredients that taste amazing together, and they also happen to be a muscle-building trifecta! You get muscle sculpting nutrients like iron (from chocolate), protein (from peanuts), and potassium (from bananas).

Serves 2

1 scoop chocolate protein powder
1 cup organic skim milk
1 ripe banana
2 tablespoons natural peanut butter
8 ice cubes
¼ teaspoon cinnamon

Combine all ingredients in a blender and blend until smooth. Add ½ to ¾ cup water for a thinner shake. Serve immediately or store in an airtight drink bottle to take to school or your office.

Nutritional Stats Per serving (serving size: 1 shake, about 1½ cups) 239 calories, 18 g protein, 16 g sugars, 26 g carbohydrates, 9 g fat (2 g saturated), 2 mg cholesterol, 4 g fiber, 166 mg sodium

SATAY PEANUT DIP

Mixing peanut butter with Greek yogurt adds a wonderful fluffy texture and more protein with less fat to this savory hunger-busting dip. If you have leftover dip, try spreading it on chicken or sliced veggies to grill up something tasty and unique.

Serves 4

½ cup smooth peanut or almond butter
¼ cup plain, 2% Greek yogurt
1 tablespoon reduced-sodium soy sauce
2 garlic cloves, minced
2 to 4 teaspoons hot sauce (2 teaspoons for medium, 4 teaspoons for spicy)
½ pound raw green beans
4 carrots, peeled and cut into matchsticks

In a small mixing bowl combine the peanut butter, yogurt, soy sauce, garlic, and hot sauce. Serve immediately with green beans and carrot sticks or transfer to an airtight container and refrigerate for up to 3 weeks.

Nutritional Stats Per serving (serving size: 3 tablespoons dip with 1 cup veggies) 242 calories, 12 g protein, 7 g sugars, 15 g carbohydrates, 17 g fat (4 g saturated), 2 mg cholesterol, 4 g fiber, 388 mg sodium

NO-BAKE PEANUT BUTTER COCONUT TRUFFLES

These no-bake treats are filled with high-quality fats that will help you feel fuller longer and help fight inflammation.

Serves 5, makes 10 truffles

1 scoop (⅓ cup) protein powder, vanilla, chocolate, or peanut butter flavor
2 tablespoons natural peanut butter
2 tablespoons unsweetened shredded coconut, plus 1 tablespoon
   (or 1 tablespoon unsweetened cocoa powder), for rolling
2 tablespoons brown sugar
1 tablespoon coconut oil
1 teaspoon cinnamon

Place the protein powder, peanut butter, 2 tablespoons shredded coconut, brown sugar, coconut oil, and cinnamon into a small bowl and mash with the back of a spoon until a thick, dry paste starts to form.

Add in a few drops of water at a time until mixture starts to clump and becomes sticky. Using your hands, roll into ten ½-inch-diameter balls. Roll in 1 tablespoon additional coconut or cocoa powder. Store in an airtight container in the refrigerator for up to 3 days or consume immediately.

Nutritional Stats Per serving (serving size: 2 truffles) 107 calories, 5 g protein, 5 g sugars, 7g carbohydrates, 7 g fat (4 g saturated), 0 mg cholesterol, 1 g fiber, 47 mg sodium

CRUNCHY CHIA KALE CHIPS

Crunchy chia seeds make these chips rival the crispiness of your standard potato chips while delivering 100 percent more nutrition. Run out of chia? No need to run right to the store: use ground flaxseed instead.

Serves 4

One 10-ounce bunch curly kale, stems trimmed
Cooking spray
½ cup grated Parmesan cheese
¼ cup chia seeds
2 tablespoons ground flaxseed
2 eggs
½ teaspoon Chef Rocco's seasoning salt

Preheat the oven to 400°F. Rinse the kale under cold water. Dry well with paper towels or a dry dishtowel. Coat two baking sheets with cooking spray.

Place the chia seeds, Parmesan, and flaxseed on a sheet of wax paper. Mix with your fingertips.

Place the eggs in a large bowl and whisk until foamy, about 10 seconds. Dip the edges of the kale leaves into the egg, then press into the chia mixture. Transfer the kale leaves to the baking sheets, spread out so the leaves aren't touching. Coat the tops of the leaves with a layer of cooking spray.

Bake 10 to 12 minutes, until the leaves crisp. Sprinkle with the seasoning salt and serve.

Nutritional Stats Per serving (serving size: 1½ cups chips) 203 calories, 12 g protein, 2 g sugars, 15 g carbohydrates, 12 g fat (3 g saturated), 102 mg cholesterol, 8 g fiber, 277 mg sodium

GUACAMOLE

Avocado is a fruit that's in season during the winter months. It just so happens that avocado is full of skin-soothing ingredients like vitamins E and C. It also contains high amounts of potassium, a mineral that is important for hydration because it balances your body's water,.

Serves 4

3 ripe avocados, preferably Hass
1 ripe tomato, seeded and finely chopped (about 1 cup)
¼ cup red onion, minced
Juice of 2 limes (about ¼ cup)
1 jalapeño pepper, seeded and finely chopped (optional)
¼ cup fresh cilantro, minced
½ teaspoon seasoning salt
1 cucumber, cut into rounds
2 carrots, peeled and cut into matchsticks
4 celery stalks, cut into matchsticks

Place the avocados, tomato, onion, lime juice, jalapeño, cilantro, and salt in a large bowl. Use a wooden spoon to mash the ingredients together. Split into four even portions and serve immediately with the vegetables.

Nutritional Stats Per serving (serving size: ½ cup guacamole with 1 cup veggies for dipping) 219 calories, 4 g protein, 6 g sugars, 20 g carbohydrates, 16 g fat (2 g saturated), 0 mg cholesterol, 10 g fiber, 356 mg sodium

LUNCHES

EMPANADAS

Raisins mixed with olives might seem strange, but together they give this empanada recipe an irresistible sweet and salty flavor, which you'll find in Latin fare.

Serves 4

1 tablespoon olive oil
1 head broccoli, cut into small florets (about 4 cups)
½ red onion, thinly sliced
½ cup pitted olives, such as kalamata

¼ cup raisins

1 teaspoon dried thyme

1 pound whole wheat pizza dough, defrosted, cut into quarters

½ cup grated cheddar cheese

Preheat oven to 400°F. Heat a large skillet over medium heat. Put in the olive oil, broccoli, onion, olives, raisins, and thyme. Cook 3 to 4 minutes, stirring occasionally, until the broccoli starts to brown and soften. Reduce the heat to low and add a few tablespoons of water. Cover and cook 1 minute more, until the broccoli is tender. Turn off the heat and let cool while you prepare the dough.

Roll the dough out into 4-inch-diameter disks, or stretch the dough out with your hands. Set out two baking dishes (or ungreased baking sheet) and place the disks a few inches apart. Place ¼ cup of the cheese on each disk. Divide the broccoli mixture between the four disks and pinch–fold over one of the edges to make a half-moon shape. Pinch the edges shut with your fingers and bake 10 to 12 minutes, until the dough is cooked through and brown around the edges. Cool 5 minutes before serving.

Nutritional Stats Per serving (serving size: 1 large empanada) 442 calories, 15 g protein, 12 g sugars, 66 g carbohydrates, 15 g fat (4 g saturated), 15 mg cholesterol, 7 g fiber, 742 mg sodium

Chef's Notes: To save time on prep, buy broccoli florets already cut up in your produce aisle and buy pre-grated cheese.

BURRITOS

Take-out bean burritos or ones that you find when you stop off at the gas station might be okay with calories, but their sodium levels are off the charts: 1,200 mg or more. Make this version with a much lower sodium count that will decrease as you go through the phases.

Serves 4

1 tablespoon olive oil

½ pound ground turkey

1 tablespoon chili powder, mild or hot

1 teaspoon ground cumin

¼ yellow or red onion, finely chopped (about ¼ cup)

2 garlic cloves, minced

1 cup canned no-salt-added diced tomatoes

OR ½ recipe of taco meat from Turkey Tacos (page 259)
1 red or green bell pepper, chopped
1 cup canned low-sodium black beans, drained and well rinsed
Four 9-inch whole wheat wraps (around 160 calories apiece)
½ cup grated mozzarella or cheddar cheese

Heat a large stockpot over medium heat. Put in the olive oil and turkey. Sear 1 to 2 minutes without stirring. Sprinkle the chili powder and cumin over the meat. Scatter the onion and garlic around the turkey and cook 2 to 3 minutes more, stirring once or twice to break up the meat.

Add the tomatoes, bell pepper, and black beans and cook 4 to 5 minutes, until a thick sauce forms. Set out four wraps and divide the meat mixture between them. Top each with 2 tablespoons of the grated cheese. Roll up the wraps, cover in aluminum foil, and warm in the oven or toaster oven for 4 to 5 minutes at 400°F. Serve immediately.

Nutritional Stats Per serving (serving size: 1 stuffed burrito) 405 calories, 24 g protein, 5 g sugars, 43 g carbohydrates, 18 g fat (4 g saturated), 47 mg cholesterol, 11 g fiber, 819 mg sodium

Chef's Note: Whip up a double portion of these, and freeze individually in aluminum foil and ziplock bags for breakfast or lunch on the go. Just reheat in a microwave or remove the bag and reheat in foil directly in a toaster oven.

CALZONE

Calzones aren't just for grown-ups. Make them mini-size to pop into lunch boxes. Just cut the dough into eight portions instead of four. Chop the veggies a bit finely, divide among the dough portions, and top with cheese and sauce. Bake 2 to 3 minutes less than the larger calzone.

Serves 4

1 pound defrosted whole wheat pizza dough, cut into quarters
1 cup low-sodium marinara sauce
1 cup grated mozzarella cheese
2 cups chopped spinach leaves or broccoli florets
1 red bell pepper, sliced
½ cup chopped olives

Preheat oven to 400°F. Roll the dough out into 4-inch-diameter disks, or stretch the dough out with your hands. Set out two baking dishes (or ungreased baking sheets) and place the disks a few inches apart. Spread ¼ cup of the marinara over each disk.

Place ¼ cup of the cheese on each disk. Divide the spinach or broccoli, bell pepper, and olives among the four disks and pinch–fold over one of the edges to make a half-moon shape. Pinch the edges shut with your fingers and bake 10 to 12 minutes, until the dough is cooked through and brown around the edges. Let cool 5 minutes before serving.

Nutritional Stats Per serving (serving size: 1 calzone or 2 minis) 394 calories, 18 g protein, 9 g sugars, 59 g carbohydrates, 9 g fat (2 g saturated), 10 mg cholesterol, 6 g fiber, 794 mg sodium

SLOPPY JOES

Forget the sloppy-joe mix that comes in a can. It has double the amount of salt per cup and doesn't taste nearly as good as this one that you can prep during the weekend and enjoy throughout the week.

Serves 4

Sloppy Joes
1 tablespoon olive oil
1 pound ground turkey
2 tablespoons chili powder, mild or hot
2 teaspoons ground cumin
½ yellow or red onion, finely chopped
3 garlic cloves, minced
3 ounces canned tomato paste
OR 1 recipe of taco meat from Turkey Tacos (page 259)
1 green or red bell pepper, chopped
1 tablespoon vinegar, white or balsamic
4 whole wheat 100-calorie sandwich flats

Coleslaw
4 cups sliced cabbage
2 carrots, shredded
½ cup plain, 2% yogurt
¼ cup olive oil–based mayonnaise
1 tablespoon vinegar, any kind
½ teaspoon Old Bay or seasoning salt

To make the sloppy joes: Heat a large stockpot over medium heat. Put in the olive oil and turkey. Sear 1 to 2 minutes without stirring. Sprinkle the chili powder and cumin over the meat. Scatter the onion and garlic around the turkey and cook 2 to 3 minutes more, stirring once or twice to break up the meat. Add the tomato paste and cook 1 minute more, stirring once or twice until the mixture becomes fragrant.

Add ½ cup water, the bell pepper, and the vinegar and cook 4 to 5 minutes, until a thick sauce forms. Set out the buns and divide the meat mixture among them.

To make the coleslaw: Place the cabbage, carrots, yogurt, mayonnaise, vinegar, and Old Bay or seasoning salt in a large bowl and toss well. Serve immediately with the sloppy joes.

> **Nutritional Stats** Per serving (serving size: 1 sloppy joe with 1 heaping cup coleslaw) 458 calories, 33 g protein, 14 g sugars, 39 g carbohydrates, 21 g fat (4 g saturated), 91 mg cholesterol, 11 g fiber, 728 mg sodium

LEMON PEPPER CHICKEN VEGGIE BOWL

Black pepper grows in clusters on incredibly high vines and historically is one of the world's most popular spices. Excellent for digestion, black pepper contains manganese,[31] which is important for blood sugar control.

Serves 4

1 cup instant brown rice, cooked according to package instructions
2 tablespoons olive oil
1 pound boneless, skinless chicken breast, cut into 1-inch-wide chunks
1 head broccoli, cut into florets (about 4 cups)
½ teaspoon freshly ground black pepper
½ teaspoon garlic or onion powder (salt-free)
Zest and juice of 1 lemon
2 tablespoons reduced-sodium soy sauce
1 red or green bell pepper, chopped
1 small cucumber or zucchini, diced

Prepare the rice and set aside. Heat a large skillet over medium-high heat. Put in the olive oil, chicken, broccoli, black pepper, and garlic or onion powder. Cook 5 to 7 minutes, stirring often, until the chicken browns and is cooked through.

Turn the heat off and add the lemon zest and juice, and the soy sauce. Toss to coat.

Divide the rice, red or green bell pepper, and cucumber or zucchini among four bowls and top with the chicken. Serve immediately.

Nutritional Stats Per serving (serving size: 3 cups) 423 calories, 32 g protein, 5 g sugars, 47 g carbohydrates, 11 g fat (2 g saturated), 72 mg cholesterol, 5 g fiber, 519 mg sodium

ITALIAN MEAT LOAF

Barbecue sauce is tasty, but most commercial brands are high in sugar and unwanted additives like HFCS, artificial colorings, and artificial flavorings. Many brands of jarred marinara are a healthier swap across the board.

Serves 4

Meat Loaf
1 pound 90–93% lean ground beef
One 5-ounce package mushrooms or 2 cups baby spinach, chopped
½ cup old-fashioned oats
½ cup grated Parmesan cheese
¼ cup fresh parsley or basil, chopped (optional)
1 egg
¼ teaspoon salt
⅛ teaspoon freshly ground black pepper
OR 1 recipe of raw meatball mixture from Spaghetti and Meatballs (page 338)
½ cup low-sodium marinara sauce

Green Beans
2 teaspoons olive oil
1 pound green beans, trimmed and cut into thirds
¼ teaspoon salt
1 lemon, cut in half
¼ cup almonds, chopped

Preheat oven to 350°F. Place the ground beef, mushrooms, oats, Parmesan, parsley or basil, egg, salt, and black pepper in a large bowl. Mix well to combine and form into a 4 x 8-inch loaf. Place in the center of a slow cooker and smooth the mixture with a spatula. Top with the marinara and cook on high about 1 hour, until firm and cooked through, or to an internal temperature of about 160°F measured on a meat thermometer.

Before you are ready to serve the meat loaf, make the green beans. Heat a large skillet over medium heat. Put in the olive oil, green beans, and salt. Cook 3 to 4 minutes, until the beans start to soften and brown. Reduce the heat to low and squeeze the lemon over the green beans. Sprinkle with the almonds and serve alongside the meat loaf.

Nutritional Stats Per serving (serving size: 2 large slices meatloaf, ¼ pound green beans) 455 calories, 37 g protein, 7 g sugars, 29 g carbohydrates, 22 g fat (8 g saturated), 128 mg cholesterol, 8 g fiber, 641 mg sodium

BUNLESS SALMON BURGERS

Who said burgers can be made only of beef? Making them from salmon means a triple threat to inflammation, a condition that can keep you from losing weight. Salmon contains three potent inflammation busters: omega-3 for your heart, special proteins that are great for the cartilage in your joints, and other compounds that can stop inflammation in your digestive tract.

Serves 4

Sweet Potato Wedges
2 medium sweet potatoes, cut into ½-inch-thick wedges
1 tablespoon olive oil
½ teaspoon Old Bay seasoning
Salmon Cakes
Two 4-ounce salmon fillets
¼ cup plain, 2% Greek yogurt
¼ cup olive oil–based mayonnaise
1 teaspoon mustard
1 egg
½ cup seasoned whole wheat bread crumbs
½ cup ground flaxseed
Cooking spray

Preheat the oven to 400°F. Cover two baking sheets with aluminum foil.

Prepare the potato wedges: Toss the sweet potatoes in a large bowl with the olive oil and seasoning. Spread the wedges on the baking sheets and bake 15 to 20 minutes, until tender.

Place the salmon fillets in an 11 x 7-inch baking dish and bake 12 to 14 minutes, until the salmon flakes when pressed with a fork. Or use leftover Orange Thyme Salmon (page 261) or Honey Glazed Salmon (page 262).

Place the cooked salmon, yogurt, mayonnaise, mustard, and egg in a large bowl. Stir with a wooden spoon, breaking up the salmon as you go. Add half the bread crumbs and gently stir to combine. Place the remaining bread crumbs and the flaxseed on a large plate. Mix with your fingertips to combine. Form the salmon mixture into four 4-inch patties and dip into the bread crumb mixture.

Coat a large skillet with cooking spray and place over medium heat. Add the salmon burgers and cook 2 to 3 minutes, turning once or twice, until both sides have browned. Transfer the burgers to plates and serve immediately with the potato wedges.

Nutritional Stats Per serving (serving size: 1 large salmon cake and about 4 ounces potato wedges) 445 calories, 20 g protein, 5 g sugars, 39 g carbohydrates, 24 g fat (4 g saturated), 37 mg cholesterol, 7 g fiber, 428 mg sodium

DINNERS

TURKEY TACOS

Canned chipotle peppers are the cure for plain old boring tacos. You can find the chipotles online or in most grocery stores that carry Mexican food products. Each can contains about eight peppers, so pack the peppers in little snack bags and toss into your freezer to use whenever you're craving smoky with a hint of heat.

Serves 4

Taco Meat
Cooking spray
1 pound ground turkey
2 tablespoons chili powder, mild or hot
2 teaspoons ground cumin
¼ teaspoon salt
½ yellow or red onion, finely chopped
3 garlic cloves, minced
3 ounces canned tomato paste
One 15-ounce can diced tomatoes

Toppings

12 corn taco shells or small corn tortillas

½ cup shredded mozzarella or cheddar cheese

1½ cups chopped baby spinach or baby kale

Coat a large skillet with cooking spray and place it over medium heat. Add the turkey. Cook 2 to 3 minutes without stirring, to allow the turkey to brown. Add the chili powder, cumin, and salt. Stir once or twice to break up the meat. Add the onion and garlic and cook 1 minute more, until the spices become fragrant,and the onion starts to soften.

Add the tomato paste and the canned tomatoes, and cook 2 to 3 minutes more, stirring occasionally, until the mixture becomes thick. Divide the meat among the 12 taco shells or tortillas and sprinkle with the cheese and baby spinach or kale. Serve immediately.

Nutritional Stats Per Serving (Serving size: 3 filled tacos) 445 calories, 32 g protein, 7 g sugars, 39 g carbohydrates, 20 g fat (8 g saturated), 88 mg cholesterol, 6 g fiber, 877 mg sodium

Chef's Tip: To make these vegetarian, don't use turkey. Instead add two 15-ounce cans drained black beans or chickpeas and ½ teaspoon fennel seeds for added flavor.

MINESTRONE

Soups are not only a great low-calorie way to fill you up, but also an easy sell when it comes to getting more veggies into yourself or into your family. If you ever find yourself at the bottom of the pot with soup and want to extend the portions, just add a handful of greens like baby spinach, kale, or beets, and a drizzle of water, before reheating.

Serves 8

3 tablespoons olive oil

4 carrots, peeled and thinly sliced

1 red onion, diced

4 celery stalks, thinly sliced

4 cloves garlic, minced

Two 32-ounce containers low-sodium chicken or vegetable broth

One 15-ounce can diced tomatoes

1 cup whole wheat or whole-grain pasta, such as mini penne or spirals

Two 15-ounce cans low-sodium beans, any variety

4 cups baby spinach

1 cup grated Parmesan cheese

Warm the olive oil in a large stockpot over medium heat. Add the carrots, onion, celery, and garlic. Cook 3 to 4 minutes, stirring often, until the vegetables start to soften. Add the chicken broth, diced tomatoes, and pasta along with 2 cups of water. Bring to a simmer, then reduce to low heat. Simmer 15 to 20 minutes, until the pasta is tender.

Add the beans and spinach and cook 1 minute more until the beans are warmed through and the spinach is wilted. Sprinkle with the Parmesan and serve immediately.

Nutritional Stats Per serving (serving size: 3 cups) 323 calories, 18 g protein, 8 g sugars, 44 g carbohydrates, 9 g fat (3 g saturated), 9 mg cholesterol, 10 g fiber, 574 mg sodium

ORANGE THYME SALMON

Fresh slices of whole orange add sweet flavor without the loads of calories and carbs that you'll find in orange juice. To save on salmon, buy it in bulk or buy a whole side of salmon and cut it into smaller fillets using poultry shears.

Serves 4

Four 4-ounce salmon fillets, skin on
4 teaspoons tomato paste
4 teaspoons chipotle peppers in adobo sauce, chopped (optional)
2 small oranges, cut into 12 slices
1 teaspoon fresh or dried thyme
1 tablespoon olive oil
12 ounces frozen sweet potato fries

Preheat oven to 400°F. Place the salmon in a 7 x 11-inch baking dish, skin side down. Place the tomato paste and chipotles in a small bowl and mix with a spoon. Spread 2 teaspoons of the tomato mixture over the top of each piece of salmon.

Arrange 3 orange slices over each piece of salmon and sprinkle with the dried thyme. Drizzle with olive oil and bake 14 to 16 minutes, until the salmon is cooked through.

While the salmon is cooking, bake the sweet potato fries according to the package instructions. Serve the salmon with the fries.

Nutritional Stats Per serving (serving size: one 4-ounce piece of salmon, three ounces sweet potato fries) 435 calories, 25 g protein, 7 g sugars, 32 g carbohydrates, 19 g fat (4 g saturated), 62 mg cholesterol, 5 g fiber, 353 mg sodium

HONEY GLAZED SALMON

Together, salmon and broccoli make a one-two punch when it comes to nutrients, because they have several "core" antioxidants that are body beautiful. Salmon is rich in omega-3s, great for everything from disease prevention to keeping your brain healthy, and broccoli is rich in sulfur-based antioxidants that are the key to liver detox.

Serves 4

Four 4-ounce salmon fillets, skin on
3 tablespoons honey
2 tablespoons low-sodium soy sauce
2 teaspoons ginger powder or finely minced gingerroot
1 clove garlic, minced
1 tablespoon olive oil
1 head broccoli, cut into florets (about 4 cups)
¼ teaspoon Old Bay or Chef Rocco's (page 344) seasoning salt
½ cup whole wheat couscous

Preheat oven to 400°F. Place the salmon fillets in a 7 x 11-inch baking dish, skin side down. Place the honey, soy sauce, ginger, and garlic in a small bowl and whisk well to combine. Drizzle the mixture over the salmon and transfer to a low rack in the oven. Bake 14 to 16 minutes, until the salmon is cooked through, but still slightly pink in the center.

While the salmon is baking, prepare the broccoli. Place a skillet over medium-high heat and put in the oil. Add the broccoli florets and sprinkle with the seasoning salt. Cook 2 to 3 minutes, stirring often, until the broccoli starts to brown. Turn the heat to low and add the couscous along with 2 cups of water. Cover and cook an additional 3 to 4 minutes, until the broccoli is fork-tender and the couscous is cooked through. Serve immediately with the salmon.

Nutritional Stats Per serving (serving size: 1 salmon fillet, 1½ cups broccoli side dish) 436 calories, 30 g protein, 15 g sugars, 38 g carbohydrates, 19 g fat (4 g saturated), 62 mg cholesterol, 4 g fiber, 488 mg sodium

Chef's Notes: Old Bay Seasoning comes with 30 percent less sodium for sodium-restricted diets. If you can't find it, Konriko Chipotle (or Jalapeño) All Purpose Seasoning is also a good choice.

CHICKEN PEANUT SATAY

Satay is an Indonesian delight: spiced meat grilled on skewers and served with a tangy peanut sauce. Peanuts are delicious in savory dishes and can boost the protein content. In fact, they are higher in protein compared with tree nuts and are a part of the legume family like beans.

Serves 4

4 boneless, skinless chicken breasts (about ¾ pound)
16 bamboo skewers
½ teaspoon chili powder
Cooking spray
⅓ cup smooth peanut or almond butter
¼ cup plain, 2% Greek yogurt
2 tablespoons reduced-sodium soy sauce
2 garlic cloves, minced
2 to 4 teaspoons hot sauce (2 teaspoons for medium, 4 teaspoons for spicy)
1 large zucchini, cut into 1-inch pieces
½ pound green beans
4 ounces whole wheat spaghetti, cooked according to the package directions

Cut each chicken breast lengthwise into 4 strips (for a total of 16 strips). Thread the chicken onto bamboo skewers. Season the chicken skewers on both sides with the chili powder. Spray a skillet or grill pan with the cooking spray. Heat over medium-high heat. Place the chicken skewers in the pan and cook for 3 to 4 minutes per side, for a total of 6 to 8 minutes, until the chicken is cooked through. Remove from heat and place the chicken on serving plates.

In a small mixing bowl combine the peanut butter, yogurt, soy sauce, garlic, and hot sauce. Set aside.

Using the same skillet or grill pan, coat again with cooking spray and place over medium-high heat. Toss in the zucchini and green beans and cook for 5 to 7 minutes, turning once halfway through the cooking time, until tender. Mix the vegetables with the pasta and peanut sauce. Serve immediately with the chicken skewers.

Nutritional Stats Per serving (serving size: 4 chicken skewers, plus pasta medley) 414 calories, 41 g protein, 7 g sugars, 33 g carbohydrates, 15 g fat (3 g saturated), 83 mg cholesterol, 3 g fiber, 629 mg sodium

Chef's Note: Sriracha, a garlicky Thai hot sauce, is definitely our hot sauce of choice! Shop for the Huy Fong Foods brand, which is the large clear plastic bottle adorned with a rooster. You'll find it in the aisle that displays condiments and hot sauces.

COCONUT SHRIMP

Coconut sounds like a decadent food reserved only for sweets, but when you enjoy the unsweetened flaked variety, you're getting a low-carb food that contains anti-inflammatory fats plus natural fiber that also helps to keep you feeling full. Don't worry about the saturated fat here; since it comes from coconut, it won't be hard on your heart.

Serves 4

1½ cups unsweetened, flaked coconut
½ cup old-fashioned oats
¼ teaspoon seasoning salt
1 egg
1 pound medium peeled, deveined shrimp (about 22 per pound)
Cooking spray
1 pound romaine lettuce, chopped
2 Hass avocados, diced
1 lime, cut into 4 wedges

Preheat the oven to 400°F. Place the coconut on a plate. Place oats in a food processor or coffee grinder along with seasoning salt and process until flour forms, about 30 seconds. Transfer to a plate.

Place the egg in a shallow bowl along with 1 tablespoon water and whisk. Working with one shrimp at a time, dip each shrimp in the oat mixture and then dredge in the egg. Press into the coconut and transfer to an ungreased cookie sheet. Repeat with remaining shrimp. Coat the tops of the shrimp with a layer of cooking spray and bake on a lower rack 12 to 14 minutes, until the coating is crispy and the shrimp are cooked through.

Divide the romaine among four plates and top with ½ diced avocado each. Serve the shrimp immediately over lettuce, about 5 to 6 shrimp per plate, with a lime wedge.

Nutritional Stats Per serving (serving size: 2 cups salad with 5 to 6 shrimp) 367 calories, 21 g protein, 3 g sugars, 21 g carbohydrates, 24 g fat (11 g saturated), 189 mg cholesterol, 10 g fiber, 722 mg sodium

COD TACOS

You don't have to wait for the dream trip to Mexico—you can have these flaky fish tacos with south-of-the-border flavors anytime. Make a double recipe of the unique cilantro pesto to serve as a flavoring for cauliflower mash or to whisk into your scrambled eggs.

Serves 4

2 cups baby spinach
2 cups cilantro leaves
¼ cup feta cheese
2 tablespoons olive oil
¼ teaspoon salt
Four 4-ounce cod fillets
OR leftover baked cod (page 342)
2 cups napa or savoy cabbage, thinly sliced
Juice of 1 lime
¼ teaspoon salt
Eight 6-inch whole wheat flour tortillas

Preheat oven to 400°F. To make the pesto, place the spinach, cilantro, feta, olive oil, and salt in a food processor. Process until a chunky mixture forms. Divide the pesto into four portions and spread over each piece of fish in a baking dish. Bake 18 to 20 minutes, until the fish flakes when pressed with a fork.

Combine the cabbage, lime juice, and salt. Toss well. Break cooked cod into pieces. Layer half a cod fillet in each tortilla, with ¼ cup of the cabbage mixture. Serve immediately.

Nutritional Stats Per serving (serving size: 2 tacos) 350 calories, 29 g protein, 1 g sugars, 30 g carbohydrates, 15 g fat (4 g saturated), 65 mg cholesterol, 5 g fiber, 693 mg sodium

SWEET POTATO STUFFER

Sweet potatoes not only are low in calories but make the perfect superfood base, rich in vitamin A, vitamin C, and pantothenic acid (also known as vitamin B_5), a crucial nutrient that we need to process fats, carbohydrates, or proteins for energy.

Serves 4

4 sweet potatoes or yams
1 cup canned black beans, drained and well rinsed

½ cup salsa
2 tablespoons olive oil
4 tablespoons sour cream

Poke the potatoes a few times with a fork. Wrap in paper towels and place on a micro-waveable dish. Cook on high for 3 to 4 minutes, then turn potatoes over. Cook on high 4 additional minutes, then—using a dishtowel to handle them—gently squeeze to test for doneness. Microwave an additional minute if they are not soft to the touch.

When the potatoes are cool enough to handle, cut them in half lengthwise. Scoop out the flesh and transfer to a bowl. Place the potato shells on a baking sheet or toaster oven tray. Add the black beans, salsa, and olive oil to the bowl with the sweet potato flesh. With a wooden spoon, mash the sweet potatoes with the beans until a chunky mixture forms.

Transfer the sweet potato mixture back into the shells and microwave, covered, on low for 20 to 30 seconds. Top with sour cream and serve immediately.

Nutritional Stats Per serving (serving size: 1 stuffed sweet potato) 370 calories, 8 g protein, 14 g sugars, 68 g carbohydrates, 9 g fat (2 g saturated), 6 mg cholesterol, 12 g fiber, 598 mg sodium

DESSERTS

BAKED APPLES

Warning! The soothing smell of these baked apples will trigger childhood memories of homemade apple pie. But no need to nosh on a calorie-dense deep-dish pie: these lean apples have the same delicious cinnamon scent and flavor.

Serves 4

¼ cup brown sugar (or 3 teaspoons of stevia)
¼ cup finely chopped walnuts
2 tablespoons olive oil
1 teaspoon cinnamon
4 apples, any variety, cut into halves

In a large bowl, mix together the brown sugar, walnuts, olive oil, and cinnamon. Set aside. Using a grapefruit spoon that has sharp edges or a melon baller or a small paring knife, remove the core and seeds from the apple halves.

Fill the apples with the walnut mixture and place them in a slow cooker. Pour 2 table-spoons of water around the apples. Set the slow cooker on high heat and cook 2 to 2½ hours until the apples are soft and begin to collapse. Serve immediately.

Nutritional Stats Per serving (serving size: 1 baked apple) 236 calories, 1 g protein, 27 g sugars, 34 g carbohydrates, 11 g fat (1 g saturated), 0 mg cholesterol, 5 g fiber, 4 mg sodium

Chef's Note: Want to make these even more flavorful without adding calories? Add 1 tea-spoon of vanilla or almond extract to the nut mixture or add 1 teaspoon of freshly zested citrus peel.

Substitutions: If you don't want to use walnuts, you could use pecans or go nut-free by substituting ¼ cup chopped raisins, prunes, or granola!

BERRY DELICIOUS FROZEN YOGURT POPS

Probiotic[32] cultured foods like yogurt not only can fight your cravings for sugar but also can boost your digestion, smooth your skin, and potentially ward off diabetes. The cultures don't die when you freeze them—this dessert is a tasty way to get more probiotics in your meals.

Serves 8

    1 cup organic skim milk
    1 cup mixed berries, such as raspberries, blueberries, or blackberries
    ½ cup plain, 2% Greek yogurt or plain kefir
    ⅓ cup protein powder
    ¼ tablespoon brown sugar or honey (or ¼ teaspoon stevia)
    2 tablespoons chopped nuts, such as walnuts or almonds
    1 teaspoon vanilla extract
    ½ teaspoon cinnamon
    8 ice cubes

Place all ingredients in a blender and process until smooth. Transfer to eight 2-ounce Popsicle molds and freeze according to the manufacturer's instructions, at least 4 hours. Rinse the mold under hot running water for 20 seconds to unmold, then serve.

Nutritional Stats Per serving (serving size: 1 Popsicle) 71 calories, 5 g protein, 8 g sugars, 10 g carbohydrates, 2 g fat (0 g saturated), 2 mg cholesterol, 2 g fiber, 28 mg sodium

BANANAS FOSTER PARFAIT

This healthier version of bananas Foster is served over sweetened high-protein Greek yogurt in place of vanilla ice cream. As you go through the phases, it will lighten in sugar and calories but still have the same great flavors.

Serves 4

Two 7-ounce containers plain, 2% Greek yogurt
4 tablespoons brown sugar (or 1 teaspoon stevia)
1 teaspoon vanilla extract
1 tablespoon olive oil
2 ripe bananas, thinly sliced
½ teaspoon rum extract (optional)

Place the yogurt, half the brown sugar, and the vanilla in a small bowl. Mix well. Set aside.

Warm the olive oil in a large skillet over medium heat. Add the banana slices and remaining brown sugar. Cook 2 to 3 minutes, turning occasionally with a metal spatula until the bananas brown. Add the rum extract if using. Reduce the heat to low and cook 1 to 2 minutes more, stirring often, until the bananas soften.

Divide the yogurt mixture among four parfait glasses and spoon over the cooked bananas. Serve immediately.

Nutritional Stats Per serving (serving size: 1 cup) 185 calories, 9 g protein, 20 g sugars, 26 g carbohydrates, 6 g fat (2 g saturated), 7 mg cholesterol, 1 g fiber, 31 mg sodium

20-DAY MEAL PLAN: ORANGE

This phase may not seem very different from your experience with the yellow level, and that's by design. As I've said over and over, there's no sense in trying to correct every single bad dietary habit you have in one fell swoop. Making small changes gradually, to move away from your old way of eating will help your palate adjust in a way that makes it easy to keep to the plan.

Once you have the right foods in the fridge and pantry, it's time to get into the meal plans. Like the yellow plan, the orange plan is a seven-day menu complete with breakfasts, snacks, lunches, dinners, and desserts, to be repeated each week. You'll find new variations on dishes you're already used to making and a few new recipes to keep things interesting and to add to your cooking mastery.

Finally, we'll get into the recipes, which are organized by meal!

SHOPPING LIST: ORANGE

Time to go leaner, cleaner, and greener. The foods at the orange level help you to step up your protein consumption while cleaning up your carb choices. Both of these things help to slow digestion a bit, so that you are less likely to store body fat. Make sure you grab this list before heading out to shop for this level, or download the lists at 20minutebody.com.

WEEK 1

DAIRY

½ gallon unsweetened, plain coconut milk

2 dozen eggs

8 ounces crumbled feta cheese

16 ounces shredded mozzarella or cheddar cheese

Two 5-ounce containers plain, 2% Greek yogurt

One 8-ounce container sour cream

½ cup grated Parmesan cheese

PRODUCE

Two 10-ounce bunches kale

3 pounds baby spinach

1 pound romaine lettuce leaves

1 head savoy or green cabbage

2 heads broccoli

1 bag carrots

1 bunch asparagus

1 bag celery

1½ pounds mushrooms, such as button or cremini

6 yellow or red onions

1 head garlic

4 large sweet potatoes

6 avocados, preferably Hass

3 medium tomatoes

2 red bell peppers

2 green bell peppers

1 small cucumber or zucchini

1 pound green beans

6 limes

3 lemons

2 jalapeño peppers

4 apples, any variety

3 cups fresh berries, such as raspberries or blueberries

1 pear

1 bunch fresh basil or parsley

1 bunch fresh mint

1 bunch fresh cilantro

MEAT, POULTRY, AND FISH

1 pound cubed beef stew meat

3 pounds ground turkey

3 pounds boneless, skinless chicken breasts (about 3 large or 4 small)

2 pounds 90–93% lean ground beef

2 pounds cod fillets

1 pound salmon fillets, skin on

FROZEN

One 8-ounce bag frozen blueberries

1 pound frozen whole wheat pizza dough

GRAINS AND DRY GROCERIES

4 small whole wheat buns (about 100 calories apiece)

8 slices whole-grain or whole wheat bread

8 hard corn taco shells

One 26-ounce bag or box whole-grain pancake mix

One 15-ounce container vanilla protein powder

4 small (6-inch) whole wheat pitas, cut in half

4 whole wheat 100-calorie sandwich flats

Four 9-inch whole wheat wraps (around 160 calories apiece)

8 ounces whole wheat spaghetti or angel hair pasta

OILS, CONDIMENTS, SPICES

One 5-ounce can olive oil cooking spray

JARRED AND CANNED GOODS

1 jar almond butter

One 26-ounce jar low-sodium marinara sauce

Two 32-ounce container low-sodium chicken broth

Three 15-ounce no-salt added diced tomatoes

Two 5-ounce cans tomato paste

One 7-ounce can chipotle peppers in adobe sauce

One 14-ounce box instant brown rice

One 12 ounce jar honey

One 4-ounce bar 70% cocoa

One 15-ounce can low-sodium beans, any variety

One 42-ounce container old-fashioned oats

One 14-ounce jar coconut oil

Three 15-ounce cans low-sodium garbanzo or kidney beans

One 15-ounce can low-sodium black beans

One 10-ounce container black olives

One 20-ounce bottle ketchup (optional)

One 4-ounce box stevia

One 15-ounce jar salsa

One 14-ounce box instant brown rice

One 12-ounce package quinoa

One 5-ounce container almonds

WEEK 2

PRODUCE

4½ pounds baby spinach

Three 10-ounce bunches kale

2 heads cabbage, such as napa or savoy

2 heads broccoli

2 bunches asparagus

1 pound green beans

1 bag carrots

2 bags celery

1 red or orange bell pepper

3 green or red bell peppers

1 small cucumber or zucchini

One 5-ounce package mushrooms

6 sweet potatoes or yams (about 2¼ pounds)

5 red or yellow onions

1 head garlic

3 tomatoes

7 avocados, preferably Hass

2 jalapeño peppers (optional)

1 bunch fresh basil

1 bunch fresh cilantro

1 bunch fresh mint

1 pear

7 limes

1 lemon

4 apples, any variety

4 cups fresh berries, such as raspberries or blueberries

MEAT, POULTRY, AND FISH

1 pound cubed beef stew meat

3 pounds ground turkey

3 pounds boneless, skinless chicken breasts

2 pounds 90–93% lean ground beef

1 pound cod fillets

1 pound salmon fillets, skin on

DAIRY

1/2 gallon plain, unsweetened coconut milk

2 dozen eggs

Two 5-ounce containers plain, 2% Greek yogurt

8 ounces grated mozzarella or cheddar cheese

One 8-ounce container sour cream

1/2 cup grated Parmesan cheese

4 ounces feta cheese

FROZEN

8 ounces frozen blueberries

GRAINS AND DRY GROCERIES

Four 9-inch whole wheat wraps (around 160 calories apiece)

4 whole wheat 100-calorie sandwich flats

4 small whole wheat buns (about 100 calories apiece)

4 small (6-inch) whole wheat pitas

8 slices whole-grain or whole wheat bread

8 hard corn taco shells

One 26-ounce container whole-grain pancake mix

One 14-ounce box instant brown rice

One 12-ounce package quinoa

8 ounces rice noodles

One 12-ounce container vanilla protein powder

Two 4-ounce bars 70% cocoa

One 5-ounce container peanuts

One 5-ounce container walnuts

One 16-ounce bag chia seeds

OILS, CONDIMENTS, SPICES

One 5-ounce can olive oil cooking spray

One 25-ounce bottle olive oil

JARRED AND CANNED GOODS

Two 15-ounce cans no-salt-added diced tomatoes

One 15-ounce can beans, any variety

Three 15-ounce cans no-salt-added chickpeas

Two 15-ounce cans black beans

One 15-ounce can no-salt-added diced tomatoes

Three 5-ounce cans no-salt-added tomato paste

48 ounces low-sodium chicken broth

One 24-ounce jar low-sodium marinara sauce

One 15-ounce jar salsa

WEEK 3

PRODUCE

One 10-ounce bunch kale

1 head butter lettuce leaves

1 head cabbage, such as napa or savoy

2 pounds baby spinach

3 pounds green beans

2 heads broccoli

1 bunch asparagus

Three 5-ounce package mushrooms

1 bag celery

4 large zucchini (about 1¼ pounds)

3 red bell peppers

1 green bell pepper

1 jalapeño pepper

3 avocados

1 tomato

4 red onions

1 head garlic

One 3-inch gingerroot

4 large sweet potatoes

1 small bunch scallions

1 bunch fresh mint

1 bunch fresh parsley

1 bunch fresh cilantro

4 lemons

4 limes

1 pear

2 cups fresh berries, such as raspberries or blueberries

1 banana

20-DAY MEAL PLAN: ORANGE

MEAT, POULTRY, AND FISH

3 pounds boneless, skinless chicken breasts

3 pounds 90–93% lean ground beef

1/2 pound nitrate-free bacon

2 1/2 pounds medium peeled, deveined shrimp (about 22 per pound)

2 pounds cod fillets

1 pound salmon fillets, skin on

DAIRY

1/2 gallon unsweetened, plain coconut milk or skim milk

2 dozen eggs

One 15-ounce container part-skim ricotta

16 ounces grated mozzarella cheese

1 cup grated Parmesan cheese

Two 5-ounce containers plain, 2% Greek yogurt or plain kefir

24 ounces grated cheddar cheese

4 ounces feta cheese

FROZEN

4 cups frozen berries, such as raspberries or blueberries

2 pounds frozen whole wheat pizza dough

GRAINS AND DRY GROCERIES

One 26-ounce container whole-grain pancake mix

8 slices whole-grain or whole wheat bread

8 hard corn taco shells

1 container old-fashioned oats

One 14-ounce box instant brown rice

One 12-ounce box whole wheat lasagna noodles

2 pounds whole wheat spaghetti

12 small (6-inch) whole wheat pitas

Two 8-inch whole wheat pitas (around 160 calories apiece)

2 large whole wheat tortillas

One 12-ounce container chocolate protein powder

OILS, CONDIMENTS, SPICES

One 25-ounce bottle olive oil

One 10-ounce bottle vinegar, any variety

One 2-ounce container crushed red pepper flakes

JARRED AND CANNED GOODS

One 28-ounce can diced tomatoes

One 16-ounce jar natural peanut butter

One 24-ounce jar low-sodium marinara sauce

One 5-ounce can no-salt-added tomato paste

Two 15-ounce cans chickpeas

One 15-ounce can black beans

Two 15-ounce cans low-sodium chicken or vegetable broth

One 15-ounce jar salsa

One 10-ounce jar or can pitted olives, such as kalamata

One 12-ounce container raisins

20-DAY MEAL PLAN: ORANGE

DAY 1

BREAKFAST

Pancakes

Chef's Note: You'll save leftovers to make Tuesday's snack!

LUNCH

Beef Stew

SNACK

Vanilla Spice Protein Bites

Chef's Note: Make enough to keep on hand for the week.

DINNER

Turkey Chili

Chef's Notes: Make extra turkey chili to use leftover for recipes throughout the week. Also, this is a good time to prep chicken for tomorrow's Thai Chicken Salad or Tasty Greek Chicken Salad.

DAY 2

BREAKFAST

Minty Lean and Green Shake

LUNCH

Tasty Greek Chicken Salad or Thai Chicken Salad

Chef's Note: This is made from chicken cooked on Day 1. Consult the recipe for exact directions.

SNACK

Guacamole with 1 cup veggies

DINNER

Beef Burger

DAY 3

BREAKFAST

Scrambles to Go

LUNCH

Sloppy Joes

Chef's Note: This is made from Day 1's leftover turkey chili meat. You'll need to save enough for Day 4's lunch, too.

SNACK

Peanut Avocado Snack or Vanilla Spice Bar

DINNER

Lemon Pepper Chicken Veggie Bowl

DESSERT

Baked Apples

Chef's Note: Healthier desserts help you stay the course. Use this opportunity to make enough for the remainder of the week and next week.

DAY 4

BREAKFAST

Baked Apple Parfait

Chef's Note: Remember yesterday's baked apples? Use those for this breakfast recipe.

LUNCH

Burrito

Chef's Note: This should come from Day 1's leftover turkey chili meat.

SNACK

Double Chocolate Milkshake

DINNER

Salsa Cod with Guacamole

Chef's Note: Use leftover guacamole for the snack on Thursday and leftover cod for the tacos.

DAY 5

BREAKFAST

Cinnamon Nut Breakfast

LUNCH

Sweet Potato Stuffer

SNACK

Guacamole with 1 cup veggies

DINNER

Cod Tacos

Chef's Note: Use leftover cod from Day 4's dinner.

DAY 6

BREAKFAST

Vanilla Spice Protein Bites

LUNCH

Buffalo Chicken

SNACK

Kale Chips

DINNER

Chipotle Salmon

DAY 7

BREAKFAST

French Toast

LUNCH

Pizza

SNACK

Spiced Chickpeas and Nuts

DINNER

Italian Meat Loaf

DESSERT

Double Chocolate Milkshake

DAY 8

BREAKFAST

Pancakes

Chef's Note: You'll save leftovers to make Day 10's snack!

LUNCH

Beef Stew

SNACK

Vanilla Spice Protein Bites

Chef's Note: Make enough to keep on hand for the week.

DINNER

Turkey Chili

Chef's Notes: Make extra turkey chili to use leftover for recipes through the week. Also, this is a good time to prep chicken for tomorrow's Thai Chicken Salad or Tasty Greek Chicken Salad.

DAY 9

BREAKFAST

Minty Lean and Green Shake

LUNCH

Tasty Greek Chicken Salad or Thai Chicken Salad

Chef's Note: This is made from chicken cooked on Day 8. Consult the recipe for exact directions.

SNACK

Guacamole with 1 cup veggies

DINNER

Beef Burger

DAY 10

BREAKFAST

Scrambles to Go

LUNCH

Sloppy Joes

Chef's Note: This is made from Day 8's leftover turkey chili meat. You'll need to save enough for Day 11's lunch, too.]

SNACK

Peanut Avocado Snack or Vanilla Spice Bar

DINNER

Lemon Pepper Chicken Veggie Bowl

DESSERT

Baked Apples

Chef's Note: Healthier desserts help you stay the course. Use this opportunity to make enough for the remainder of the week and next week.

DAY 11

BREAKFAST

Baked Apple Parfait

Chef's Note: Remember yesterday's baked apples? Use those for this breakfast recipe.

LUNCH

Burrito

Chef's Note: This should come from Day 8's leftover turkey chili meat.

SNACK

Double Chocolate Milkshake

DINNER

Salsa Cod with Guacamole

Chef's Note: Use leftover guacamole for the snack on Thursday and leftover cod for the tacos.

DAY 12

BREAKFAST

Cinnamon Nut Breakfast Cereal

LUNCH

Sweet Potato Stuffer

SNACK

Guacamole with 1 cup veggies

DINNER

Cod Tacos

Chef's Note: Use leftover cod from Day 11's dinner.

DAY 13

BREAKFAST

Vanilla Spice Protein Bites

LUNCH

Buffalo Chicken

SNACK

Kale Chips

DINNER

Chipotle Salmon

DAY 14

BREAKFAST
French Toast

LUNCH
Pizza

SNACK
Spiced Chickpeas and Nuts

DINNER
Italian Meat Loaf

DESSERT
Double Chocolate Milkshake

DAY 15

BREAKFAST
Pancakes

Chef's Note: You'll save leftovers to make Day 17's snack!

LUNCH
Beef Stew

SNACK
Vanilla Spice Protein Bites

Chef's Note: Make enough to keep on hand for the week.

DINNER
Turkey Chili

Chef's Notes: Make extra turkey chili to use leftover for recipes through the week. Also, this is a good time to prep chicken for tomorrow's Thai Chicken Salad or Tasty Greek Chicken Salad.

DAY 16

BREAKFAST

Minty Lean and Green Shake

LUNCH

Tasty Greek Chicken Salad or Thai
Chicken Salad

Chef's Note: This is made from
chicken cooked on Day 15. Consult
the recipe for exact directions.

SNACK

Guacamole with 1 cup veggies

DINNER

Beef Burger

DAY 17

BREAKFAST

Scrambles to Go

LUNCH

Sloppy Joes

Chef's Note: This is made from
Day 15's leftover turkey chili meat.
You'll need to save enough for Day
18's lunch, too.

SNACK

Peanut Avocado Snack or Vanilla
Spice Bar

DINNER

Lemon Pepper Chicken Veggie
Bowl

DESSERT

Baked Apples

Chef's Note: Healthier desserts
help you stay the course. Use this
opportunity to make enough for
the remainder of the week.

DAY 18

BREAKFAST

Baked Apple Parfait

Chef's Note: Remember yesterday's baked apples? Use those for this breakfast recipe.

LUNCH

Burrito

Chef's Note: This should come from Day 15's leftover turkey chili meat.

SNACK

Double Chocolate Milkshake

DINNER

Salsa Cod with Guacamole

Chef's Notes: Use leftover guacamole for the snack on Thursday and leftover cod for the tacos.

DAY 19

BREAKFAST

Cinnamon Nut Breakfast Cereal

LUNCH

Sweet Potato Stuffer

SNACK

Guacamole with 1 cup veggies

DINNER

Cod Tacos

Chef's Note: Use leftover cod from Day 18's dinner.

DAY 20

BREAKFAST
Vanilla Spice Protein Bites

LUNCH
Buffalo Chicken

SNACK
Kale Chips

DINNER
Chipotle Salmon

20-DAY RECIPES: ORANGE

You've already gotten accustomed to being in the kitchen preparing quick-and-easy meals. Now, you're just using more wholesome, body-friendly ingredients. Use these recipes to start speeding your way toward a body that refuses to hold on to body fat—one that is always satisfied, never stuffed. And again, these recipes are designed to help you get into and out of the kitchen so you can get back to your life.

BREAKFASTS

PANCAKES

Protein powder and flaxseed or chia seeds give your run-of-the-mill pancakes triple the amount of filling protein. Eating enough protein keeps hunger pangs away, and helps to anchor blood sugar. Don't toss leftover pancakes: place them in a ziplock bag and make the Spicy Peanut Avocado Snack on page 292, perfectly portable for work, school, or post-gym workout.

Serves 4, makes twelve 3-inch pancakes

¾ cup whole-grain pancake mix
⅓ cup protein powder
2 tablespoons ground flaxseed or chia seeds
¾ cup plain, unsweetened coconut milk
1 egg
1 tablespoon almond butter
Cooking spray
1 cup fresh berries, such as raspberries or blueberries
¼ cup real maple syrup

Place the pancake mix, protein powder, and ground flaxseed or chia seeds in a large bowl. Mix well with a whisk. Add the coconut milk, egg, and almond butter. Stir until just combined, about 12 turns; there will be lumps.

Coat a large skillet with cooking spray. Set over medium heat. Using a ¼-cup scoop, ladle out 4 scoops of batter, 1 inch apart. Cook 2 to 3 minutes, until bubbles start to form around the edges.

Flip and cook 2 to 3 minutes more, until the pancakes are cooked through. Transfer to a plate and repeat with remaining batter. Sprinkle with the berries and serve immediately with maple syrup.

Nutritional Stats Per serving (serving size: 3 pancakes, berries, plus 1 tablespoon syrup) 265 calories, 11 g protein, 14 sugars, 41 g carbohydrates, 7 g fat (1 g saturated), 46 mg cholesterol, 6 g fiber, 245 mg sodium

Chef's Note: Add 2 tablespoons bittersweet morsels to the batter to make a dessert "cake" for kids that isn't loaded with sugar.

FRENCH TOAST

Protein powder melts away into your egg and milk for this tasty warm breakfast and replaces protein that is lacking in coconut milk. Getting more protein-dense meals, along with plenty of anti-inflammatory foods, like berries, is a boon for your metabolic muscle.

Serves 4

1 cup plain, unsweetened coconut milk
1 egg
⅓ cup protein powder
2 tablespoons ground flaxseed
1 teaspoon vanilla extract
¼ teaspoon ground cinnamon
8 slices whole-grain or whole wheat bread
Cooking spray
1 cup fresh berries, such as raspberries or blueberries

Place the milk, egg, protein powder, flaxseed, vanilla, and cinnamon in a large, shallow bowl and whisk well. Using the tines of a fork, poke the bread several times to allow better absorption of the liquid.

Coat a large skillet with cooking spray and place it over medium heat. Dip four of the bread slices into the egg mixture and transfer to the skillet. Cook 2 to 3 minutes per side; until golden; then turn. Cook 2 to 3 minutes more, until a crisp crust has formed. Transfer to a plate and repeat with cooking spray and remaining bread. Top with berries and serve immediately.

Nutritional Stats Per serving (serving size: 2 slices French toast, plus ¼ cup berries) 301 calories, 15 g protein, 11 g sugars, 48 g carbohydrates, 4 g fat (2 g saturated), 46 mg cholesterol, 10 g fiber, 430 mg sodium

20-DAY MEAL PLAN: ORANGE

Testing Note: Most of the protein scoopers measure ⅓ cup, that's why I call for ⅓ cup in the recipe. I used Almond Breeze coconut milk and Diamond brand throughout the testing process for breakfast and desserts.

MINTY LEAN AND GREEN SHAKE

Switching from dairy milk to coconut milk is a boon for people with allergies. It's also an easy to way to cut carbs, and slim down while you sip.

Serves 2

1 cup kale
3 stalks celery
½ ripe pear, seeded
2 scoops protein powder (about ⅔ cup)
2 cups coconut milk
2 tablespoons fresh mint
1 tablespoon brown sugar
8 ice cubes

Place all the ingredients in a blender and blend until very smooth. Serve immediately.

Nutritional Stats Per serving (serving size: 1½ cups) 247 calories, 19 g protein, 18 g sugars, 29 g carbohydrates, 7 g fat (6 g saturated), 0 mg cholesterol, 5 g fiber, 189 mg sodium

SCRAMBLES TO GO

Coffee shop egg sandwiches might seem like a convenience that's also calorie conscious, but the convenience has side effects: high sodium and low fiber, meaning that your blood pressure shoots up along with your blood sugar. Opt for this easy breakfast that cooks in under 5 minutes and provides 7 grams of filling fiber.

Serves 4

Cooking spray
3 cups sliced mushrooms, asparagus pieces, or chopped spinach
6 eggs
4 egg whites or ½ cup egg whites from the carton
4 small (6-inch) whole wheat pitas, cut in half

Coat a large skillet with cooking spray. Set over high heat and add the mushrooms, asparagus, or spinach. Cook 2 to 3 minutes, stirring often, until the vegetables soften. Lower the heat to medium and carefully add another layer of the cooking spray.

Add the eggs and cook 3 to 4 minutes more, scrambling the egg mixture continuously with a fork or spatula, until soft curds form.

Divide the scrambled eggs among the pita halves and serve immediately or wrap in aluminum foil to go.

Nutritional Stats Per serving (serving size: 1 small pita stuffed with eggs) 318 calories, 21 g protein, 2 g sugars, 41 g carbohydrates, 9 g fat (3 g saturated), 279 mg cholesterol, 7 g fiber, 524 mg sodium

BAKED APPLE BREAKFAST PARFAIT

Looking for a way to zap tummy fat? Studies say that consumption of cultured dairy products like plain, low-fat yogurt may help to decrease adipose fat, especially around the midsection.

Serves 4

    8 baked apple halves
    2 cups plain, 2% Greek yogurt
    2 teaspoons stevia

Cut each baked apple half into four even strips. Place the yogurt in a small bowl and add the stevia. Stir well.

Layer ¼ cup of the yogurt mixture into four glasses, top each with two slices of the apple, repeat with remaining yogurt and apple slices, and serve.

Nutritional Stats Per serving (serving size: 1 parfait) 311 calories, 12 g protein, 32 g sugars, 40 g carbohydrates, 14 g fat (3 g saturated), 8 mg cholesterol, 5 g fiber, 37 mg sodium

20-DAY MEAL PLAN: ORANGE

CINNAMON NUT BREAKFAST CEREAL

Cutting back on sugar when you can is always a good idea, and it doesn't mean you have to cut out the flavors you love in foods. To give this cereal a "cinnamon toast" flavor, sprinkle in ¼ cup raisins and 1 teaspoon vanilla or almond extract during the last minute of cooking.

Serves 4

1 cup old-fashioned oats
½ cup quinoa, rinsed under cold running water if not prewashed (see Chef's Tip)
4 scoops protein powder (1⅓ cups)
2 teaspoons brown sugar
1 teaspoon cinnamon
¼ cup chopped nuts, such as walnuts or almonds
1 cup fresh berries, such as raspberries or blueberries

Place the oats, quinoa, protein powder, brown sugar, and cinnamon in a medium sauce-pan. Add 6½ cups of water and bring to a simmer over medium-low heat. Cover and cook 10 to 15 minutes, stirring often, until the quinoa is tender. Top with nuts and berries, and serve immediately.

Nutritional Stats Per serving (serving size: 2 cups) 325 calories, 26 g protein, 5 g sugars, 40 g carbohydrates, 10 g fat (2 g saturated), 0 mg cholesterol, 9 g fiber, 82 mg sodium

Chef's Tip: Shop for quinoa in the rice aisle of your favorite large grocery store or look for it in health food stores. If possible, buy it "prewashed" since quinoa has a natural coating that can make it taste bitter.

SNACKS

VANILLA SPICE PROTEIN BITES

Here's a clever way to cut back on sugar. Fool your nose and snack on these seemingly sweet bars that taste and smell so great because they are loaded with lots of spices and aromatic vanilla extract.

Makes 16

Cooking spray
½ cup fresh or frozen blueberries
¼ cup natural peanut butter or almond butter
2 eggs
2 teaspoons stevia
1½ cups rolled oats
4 ounces 70% cocoa, chopped
2 scoops vanilla protein powder (⅔ cup)
2 tablespoons ground flaxseed
2 tablespoons chia seeds
1 teaspoon vanilla extract
½ teaspoon cinnamon
¼ teaspoon cardamom

Preheat oven to 400F. Line an 8 x 8-inch baking dish with aluminum foil. Coat the foil with cooking spray. In a large bowl combine the blueberries, peanut butter or almond butter, eggs, and stevia. Mash with the back of a spoon.

Place the oats in a food processor and process until a chunky flour forms, about 20 pulses. Add the oats to the bowl along with the remaining ingredients.

Mash well with a fork until a thick crumbly mixture forms (this will decrease baking time), then transfer to the baking dish. Press into an even layer in the prepared pan with a rubber spatula. Bake 10 to 12 minutes, until the oats are golden and firm. Cool completely before cutting into 16 bars.

Nutritional Stats Per serving (serving size: 1 bite, 2-inch square) 158 calories, 8 g protein, 3 g sugars, 18 g carbohydrates, 8 g fat (3 g saturated), 23 mg cholesterol, 5 g fiber, 38 mg sodium

GUACAMOLE

Pack this ultra-delicious snack for the office so you won't be tempted to hit the vending machine when 3 o'clock rolls around. Skipping the chips with this guac means that you can squeeze in two whole extra servings of veggies for a lot less calories.

Serves 4

3 ripe avocados, preferably Hass
1 ripe tomato, seeded and finely chopped (about 1 cup)
¼ cup minced red onion
Juice of 2 limes (about ¼ cup)
1 jalapeño pepper, seeded and finely chopped (optional)
¼ cup fresh cilantro, minced
¼ teaspoon seasoning salt
1 cucumber, cut into rounds
2 carrots, peeled and cut into matchsticks
4 celery stalks, cut into matchsticks

Place the avocados, tomato, onion, lime juice, jalapeño (if using), cilantro, and salt in a large bowl. Use a wooden spoon to mash the ingredients together. Split into four even portions and serve immediately with the vegetables.

Nutritional Stats Per serving (serving size: ½ cup guacamole with 1 cup veggies for dipping) 219 calories, 4 g protein, 6 g sugars, 20 g carbohydrates, 16 g fat (2 g saturated), 0 mg cholesterol, 10 g fiber, 210 mg sodium

SPICY PEANUT AVOCADO SNACK

Can't get enough of this snack? Turn it into a meal by serving filled pancakes over 2 cups of your favorite salad greens per person. Prewashed greens make prep a snap—just go for power greens like baby kale, spinach, bok choy, and beet greens.

Serves 6

Leftover pancakes (page 286)
OR ¾ cup whole-grain or gluten-free pancake mix
⅓ cup protein powder
2 tablespoons ground flaxseed or chia seeds
¾ cup plain, unsweetened coconut milk
1 egg

Cooking spray
1 recipe Satay Peanut Dip (page 250)
¾ cup mashed ripe avocado

Place the pancake mix, protein powder, and flaxseed or chia seeds in a large bowl. Mix well with a whisk. Add the coconut milk and egg. Whisk well until just combined.

Coat a large skillet with cooking spray. Set over medium heat. Using a ¼ cup scoop, ladle out four scoops of batter, 1 inch apart. Cook 2 to 3 minutes until bubbles start to form around the edges. Repeat with the remaining batter, to make a total of 12 pancakes.

Set out six pancakes and divide the satay peanut dip among them. Top with the avocado and another pancake. Serve immediately or wrap in aluminum foil and keep refrigerated for up to 2 days.

Nutritional Stats Per serving (serving size: 1 pancake snack) 253 calories, 10 g protein, 5 g sugars, 27 g carbohydrates, 13 g fat (3 g saturated), 32 mg cholesterol, 4 g fiber, 255 mg sodium

DOUBLE CHOCOLATE MILKSHAKE

Getting your 25 grams of daily fiber might seem challenging but there's no need to buy a fiber supplement when you follow my plan. This dessert shake alone has 5 grams because it includes high-fiber foods like avocado that will be used throughout the plan.

Serves 2

1½ cups plain, unsweetened coconut milk
¼ ripe Hass avocado
⅓ cup protein powder
2 tablespoons unsweetened cocoa powder
3 tablespoons bittersweet chocolate chips
1 tablespoon brown sugar
1 teaspoon vanilla extract
10 ice cubes

Place all ingredients in a blender and process until smooth.

Nutritional Stats Per serving (serving size: 1 shake) 229 calories, 11 g protein, 16 g sugars, 23 g carbohydrates, 12 g fat (7 g saturated), 0 mg cholesterol, 5 g fiber, 77 mg sodium

CRUNCHY CHIA KALE CHIPS

Curly kale with frilly edges makes the best kale chips and it's the variety that's normally in your local grocery store's produce aisle. Look for firm green leaves, free of yellow spots or wilting. Always store kale in the crisper drawer in your fridge.

Serves 4

One 10-ounce bunch curly kale, stems trimmed
Cooking spray
¼ cup chia seeds
½ cup grated Parmesan cheese
2 tablespoons ground flaxseed
1 egg
3 tablespoons protein powder
½ teaspoon Chef Rocco's Seasoning Salt (page 344)

Preheat the oven to 400°F. Rinse the kale under cold water. Dry well with paper towels or a dry dishtowel. Coat two baking sheets with cooking spray.

Place the chia seeds, Parmesan, and flaxseed on a sheet of wax paper. Mix with your fingertips.

Place the egg in a large bowl along with the protein powder and 1 tablespoon water. Whisk until foamy, about 10 seconds. Dip the edges of the kale leaves into the egg, then press into the chia mixture. Transfer the kale leaves to the two baking sheets, spread out so the leaves aren't touching. Coat the tops of the leaves with a layer of cooking spray.

Bake 10 to 12 minutes, until the leaves crisp. Sprinkle with the seasoning salt and serve.

Nutritional Stats Per serving (serving size: 1½ cups chips) 198 calories, 13 g protein, 2 g sugars, 16 g carbohydrates, 11 g fat (3 g saturated), 55 mg cholesterol, 8 g fiber, 268 mg sodium

SPICED CHICKPEAS AND NUTS

Want to instantly improve some of your eating habits, like snacking mindlessly in front of the TV? It's easier than you think: just swap some TV time and go for a nighttime walk. Eat your snacks (only when hungry) at the dinner table or at your desk at work, mindfully, without working on the computer while you nosh.

Serves 6

Two 15-ounce cans chickpeas, drained and well rinsed
3 tablespoons olive oil
½ teaspoon cumin
½ teaspoon chili powder
½ teaspoon ginger
¼ teaspoon cayenne pepper
1 cup chopped walnuts

Preheat the oven to 400°F. Drain and rinse the chickpeas and lay them out on paper towels, rubbing gently to dry.

Transfer the chickpeas to a large bowl along with the olive oil and the spices. Toss well and transfer to a rimmed baking sheet, lined with aluminum foil.

Bake for 30 to 35 minutes, until the chickpeas start to brown. Add the nuts and stir well. Bake 5 additional minutes, until the nuts start to brown and the chickpeas are crisp. Serve warm, or let cool completely and store on the countertop in an airtight container for up to 5 days.

Nutritional Stats Per serving (serving size: ¾ cup) 167 calories, 7 g protein, 7 g sugars, 19 g carbohydrates, 7 g fat (1 g saturated), 0 mg cholesterol, 6 g fiber, 398 mg sodium

LUNCHES

BEEF STEW

Looking for a shortcut to slicing and dicing? Use the grated raw slaw mix that comes in a bag in place of the carrots and celery here. Cabbage is a nutrient-dense swap for celery, which doesn't have a huge vitamin load.

Serves 4

1 pound cubed beef stew meat
1 cup diced canned tomatoes
4 carrots, peeled and chopped
2 celery stalks, chopped
1 onion, chopped
2 tablespoons tomato paste
2 garlic cloves, chopped
1 teaspoon chili powder

2 cups thinly sliced baby spinach

1 cup instant brown rice, cooked according to package instructions

Place the beef, tomatoes, carrots, celery, onion, tomato paste, garlic, and chili powder in a slow cooker and stir well. Cook 3 to 3½ hours, on high heat, stirring once or twice. Sprinkle the spinach over the beef and cover to wilt, about 5 minutes. Serve immediately over rice.

Nutritional Stats Per serving (serving size: 2 cups) 415 calories, 31 g protein, 7 g sugars, 50 g carbohydrates, 10g fat (3 g saturated), 55 mg cholesterol, 5 g fiber, 302 mg sodium

Chef's Note: Grass-fed beef not only tastes better than corn-fed beef but also has a very different nutrition profile, with more omega-3s—rivaling wild salmon. To save, buy grass-fed beef from your local farmer in bulk and freeze for deliciously beefy meals to come!

Find grass-fed meats at www.americangrassfed.org/.

THAI CHICKEN SALAD

Combining several varieties of cruciferous vegetables in one meal, like cabbage and kale or cauliflower and broccoli,[33] power-charges their anticancer abilities and adds plenty of interesting texture and flavor to your plate.

Serves 4

Salad

juice of 2 limes (about ¼ cup)

2 tablespoons olive oil

2 tablespoons reduced-sodium soy sauce or fish sauce

2 tablespoons balsamic vinegar

2 large garlic cloves, minced

1 teaspoon granulated sugar

4 cups thinly sliced cabbage, such as napa or savoy

2 cups thinly sliced kale

2 cups thinly sliced spinach

1 red or orange bell pepper, thinly sliced

2 ounces rice noodles, cooked according to the package directions

¼ cup chopped peanuts

Chicken

3 boneless, skinless chicken breasts

1 teaspoon chili powder

1 tablespoon olive oil
OR chicken from Buffalo Chicken (page 300) or Chicken Peanut Satay (page 263)

Prepare the salad: In a large bowl, whisk the lime juice, olive oil, soy or fish sauce, balsamic vinegar, garlic, and sugar until smooth. Add the cabbage, kale, spinach, pepper, rice noodles, and peanuts and toss well. Set aside.

Sprinkle the chicken with the chili powder. Heat a large skillet over medium heat and put in the olive oil and the chicken. Cook 4 to 5 minutes, turning often, until the chicken is brown and cooked through. Transfer to a plate and let cool slightly before chopping into bite-size pieces. Arrange the salad on four plates, top with the chicken, and serve immediately.

Nutritional Stats Per serving (serving size: 2½ cups) 414 calories, 34 g protein, 7 g sugars, 28 g carbohydrates, 19 g fat (3 g saturated), 82 mg cholesterol, 4 g fiber, 581 mg sodium

TASTY GREEK CHICKEN SALAD

Enjoying cheese is okay when you limit the portion size, and tangy feta adds flavor and creamy texture to this filling salad. If it's in your budget, look for imported feta, since many imported brands are made with ewe's or goat's milk (rather than cow's milk), and so are high in omega-3s.

Serves 4

1 pound boneless, skinless chicken breasts (about 3 large or 4 small)
2 tablespoons coconut or olive oil
1 teaspoon oregano
1 teaspoon parsley
1 teaspoon garlic powder
1 teaspoon onion powder
1 teaspoon black pepper
½ teaspoon cinnamon
½ teaspoon nutmeg
1 pound romaine lettuce leaves, chopped
2 cups thinly sliced kale
1 cup canned low-sodium beans, such as garbanzo or kidney
½ cup crumbled feta
Juice of 1 lemon
¼ cup chopped black olives

Place the chicken, coconut or olive oil, oregano, parsley, garlic powder, onion powder, pepper, and cinnamon in a slow cooker. Toss well to coat the chicken in the spices. Set to low heat and cook 2 to 2½ hours, until the chicken is tender. Transfer the chicken to a cutting board and let cool 5 minutes.

Put the romaine and kale on a platter. Thinly slice the chicken and transfer it to the platter. Sprinkle with the beans, feta, lemon juice, and olives. Serve immediately.

Nutritional Stats Per serving (serving size: 3½ cups) 337 calories, 33 g protein, 4 g sugars, 22 g carbohydrates, 14 g fat (4 g saturated), 89 mg cholesterol, 7 g fiber, 502 mg sodium

SLOPPY JOES

Having trouble cutting back on bread? Hundred-calorie sandwich thins are a great swap for high-carb rolls because the thins have less calories and more fiber, so they help control the carb count and cravings.

Serves 4

Sloppy Joes
Cooking spray
1 tablespoon olive oil
1 pound ground turkey
2 tablespoons chili powder, mild or hot
2 teaspoons ground cumin
½ yellow or red onion, finely chopped
3 garlic cloves, minced
3 ounces canned tomato paste
OR meat from 1 recipe of Turkey Chili (page 301)
1 green or red bell pepper, chopped
1 tablespoon vinegar, white or balsamic
4 whole wheat 100-calorie sandwich flats

Coleslaw
4 cups sliced cabbage
2 carrots, shredded
½ cup plain, 2% Greek yogurt
¼ cup olive oil–based mayonnaise
1 tablespoon vinegar, any kind
¼ teaspoon Old Bay or seasoning salt

Make the sloppy joes: Coat a large stockpot with cooking spray. Place it over medium heat. Add the olive oil and turkey. Sear 1 to 2 minutes without stirring, then sprinkle the chili powder and cumin over the meat. Scatter the onion and garlic around the turkey and cook 2 to 3 minutes more, stirring once or twice to break up the meat. Add the tomato paste and cook 1 minute more, stirring once or twice, until the paste becomes fragrant.

Add ½ cup water, bell pepper, and vinegar and cook 4 to 5 minutes, until a thick sauce forms. Set out the four sandwich flats and divide the meat mixture among them.

Make the coleslaw: Place the cabbage, carrots, yogurt, mayonnaise, vinegar, and Old Bay or seasoning salt in a large bowl and toss well. Serve immediately with the sloppy joes.

Nutritional Stats Per serving (serving size: 1 sloppy joe with 1 heaping cup coleslaw) 428 calories, 33 g protein, 14 g sugars, 39 g carbohydrates, 18 g fat (4 g saturated), 91 mg cholesterol, 11 g fiber, 688 mg sodium

BURRITOS

Stock up on salt-free diced tomatoes and low-sodium beans for an easy way to snip the salt in your diet. Another simple way to cut all the bad stuff, including trans fat, tons of salt, sugar, and preservatives? Cook at home!

Serves 4

1 tablespoon olive oil
½ pound ground turkey
1 tablespoon chili powder, mild or hot
1 teaspoon ground cumin
¼ yellow or red onion, finely chopped (about ¼ cup)
2 garlic cloves, minced
1 cup canned no-salt-added diced tomatoes
OR ½ recipe of Turkey Chili (page 301)
1 red or green bell pepper, chopped
1 cup canned low-sodium black beans, drained, well rinsed
Four 9-inch whole wheat wraps (around 160 calories apiece)
¼ cup grated mozzarella or cheddar cheese

Heat a large stockpot over medium heat. Put in the olive oil and turkey. Sear 1 to 2 minutes without stirring, then sprinkle the chili powder and cumin over the meat. Scatter the onion and garlic around the turkey and cook 2 to 3 minutes more, stirring once or twice, to break up the meat.

Add the tomatoes, bell pepper, and beans, and cook 4 to 5 minutes, until a thick sauce forms. Set out four wraps and divide the meat mixture among them. Top each with 1 tablespoon of the grated cheese. Roll up the wraps, cover in aluminum foil, and warm in the oven or toaster oven for 4 to 5 minutes at 400°F. Serve immediately.

Nutritional Stats Per serving (serving size: 1 stuffed burrito) 385 calories, 22 g protein, 5 g sugars, 43 g carbohydrates, 17 g fat (3 g saturated), 44 mg cholesterol, 11 g fiber, 769 mg sodium

BUFFALO CHICKEN

Don't let blueberries take all the credit; beans are surprisingly high in antioxidant load. Beans are also a fiber all-star, so they make for a slower energy uptake compared with white processed sugars and carbs.

Serves 4

2 tablespoons olive oil
2 garlic cloves, minced
½ cup low-sodium chicken broth
¼ cup hot sauce
2 tablespoons tomato paste
2 teaspoons mild chili powder
3 skinless, boneless chicken breasts
1 head broccoli, cut into florets
4 stalks celery, cut into ½-inch pieces
One 15-ounce can no-salt-added chickpeas, rinsed and drained

Heat a small saucepan over medium heat. Put in 1 tablespoon olive oil and the garlic. Cook the garlic 1 to 2 minutes, stirring often, until fragrant. Add the chicken broth, hot sauce, tomato paste, and chili powder. Cook 2 to 3 minutes more, stirring occasionally, until the sauce thickens. Set aside.

Heat a large skillet over medium heat. Put in the remaining 1 tablespoon olive oil. Add the chicken, broccoli, and celery, and cook 3 to 4 minutes, stirring often, until the broccoli browns. Add the hot sauce mixture and the chickpeas. Cover, reduce the heat to low, and cook 1 minute more, until the sauce thickens and the chicken is cooked through. Serve immediately.

Nutritional Stats Per serving (serving size: 2½ cups) 434 calories, 41 g protein, 9 grams sugars, 39 g carbohydrates, 14 g fat (2 g saturated), 82 mg cholesterol, 9 g fiber, 411 mg sodium

PIZZA

Pizza when you're trying to lose weight? You bet. This recipe uses slow-burning fuel from whole-grain dough and an assortment of veggies to give you a flavorful but health-happy pie.

Serves 4 (2 slices per serving)

1 pound whole wheat pizza dough, defrosted, rolled out into an 8-inch disk
1 cup low-sodium marinara sauce
1½ cups grated mozzarella cheese
1 cup chopped spinach
1 red bell pepper, thinly sliced
1 cup thinly sliced mushrooms

Preheat oven to 450°F. Transfer the pizza dough onto a baking sheet or a 10-inch pizza pan. Using a spatula, spread the marinara sauce over the pizza, leaving a 1-inch border. Sprinkle with the mozzarella.

Sprinkle the spinach, bell pepper, and mushrooms over the cheese and transfer the pan to the oven. Bake 15 to 20 minutes, until the cheese is bubbly and the vegetables begin to brown. Remove from the oven and let cool 5 minutes before slicing. Cut into 8 slices and serve.

Nutritional Stats Per serving (serving size: 2 slices of pizza) 416 calories, 22 g protein, 9 g sugars, 58 g carbohydrates, 10 g fat (3 g saturated), 15 mg cholesterol, 5 g fiber, 765 mg sodium

DINNERS

TURKEY CHILI

Beans freeze beautifully, so you can use leftover beans from the can for many of the savory recipes throughout this book or anytime you want to go meatless for your meal. Just be sure they are drained and well rinsed before you transfer to ziplock bags for freezing.

Serves 6

1 tablespoon olive oil
1 pound ground turkey
2 tablespoons chili powder, mild or hot
2 teaspoons ground cumin
1 yellow or red onion, finely chopped

3 garlic cloves, minced
3 ounces canned tomato paste
One 15-ounce can no-salt diced tomatoes
32 ounces low-sodium chicken broth
2 cups baby spinach
2 cups kale, thinly sliced
1 cup canned beans, any variety, drained and well rinsed

Heat a large stockpot over medium heat. Put in the olive oil and turkey. Sear 1 to 2 minutes without stirring, then sprinkle the chili powder and cumin over the meat. Scatter the onion and garlic around the turkey and cook 2 to 3 minutes more, stirring once or twice, to break up the meat. Add the tomato paste and cook 1 minute more, stirring once or twice, until the paste becomes fragrant.

Add the diced tomatoes and cook 4 to 5 minutes more if using for Sloppy Joes (page 298) or Burritos (page 299).

Add the chicken broth, spinach, kale, and beans. Bring to a simmer over medium heat. Cook 5 to 6 minutes, until the meat is cooked through and the vegetables are tender.

Nutritional Stats Per serving (serving size: 2 cups) 228 calories, 22 g protein, 6 g sugars, 20 g carbohydrates, 9 g fat (3 g saturated), 53 mg cholesterol, 7 g fiber, 640 mg sodium

BEEF BURGERS WITH SWEET POTATO CHIPS

Looking for a rainy-day project for your kids? Have them help make sweet potato chips. You slice them, then let the kids bake them in a toaster oven. Munching along the way is a must.

Serves 4

Burgers
1 pound 90–93% lean ground beef
One 5-ounce package mushrooms or 2 cups baby spinach, chopped
¼ teaspoon salt or seasoning salt
⅛ teaspoon freshly ground black pepper
OR 1 recipe of meatball meat mixture from Spaghetti and Meatballs (page 338)
Cooking spray
4 small whole wheat buns (about 100 calories apiece)
1 medium tomato, sliced
1 small red onion, sliced

1 cup baby spinach

4 teaspoons ketchup (optional)

Sweet Potato Chips

4 large sweet potatoes, skin on

1 tablespoon olive oil

½ teaspoon seasoning salt

Place the beef, mushrooms or spinach, salt, and black pepper in a bowl. Mix well with your hands, form into four patties, and place on a plate.

Preheat oven to 375°F. Heat an ovenproof skillet or a grill pan over medium-high heat. Coat the burgers with the spray, then place them on the grill pan or skillet. Cook the burgers for 3 to 4 minutes per side.

Transfer to the oven and bake 10 minutes for medium rare and 15 minutes for medium.

Meanwhile make the chips. Wash the sweet potatoes under cold running water, do not peel. Dry well with a dishtowel. Using a vegetable slicer, or Japanese mandolin (page 113), cut the potatoes into ⅛-inch slices. Transfer to a large bowl along with the olive oil and seasoning salt, and toss well. Spread the chips out on ungreased baking sheets and bake 8 to 10 minutes, until they are crisp and start to brown.

Place each burger on a bun and top with a quarter of the tomato slices, onion slices, baby spinach, and ketchup (if using). Serve immediately with a side of sweet potato chips.

Nutritional Stats Per serving (serving size: 1 quarter-pound burger with 20 chips) 420 calories, 32 g protein, 9 g sugars, 39 g carbohydrates, 16 g fat (5 g saturated), 74 mg cholesterol, 8 g fiber, 580 mg sodium

LEMON PEPPER CHICKEN VEGGIE BOWL

Have leftover cooked brown rice? Here's a great way to use it. To save time, cook a double batch of brown rice and let cool to room temperature. Pack in ziplock bags and freeze for fast weekday meals.

Serves 4

¾ cup instant brown rice, cooked according to the package instructions

1 tablespoon olive oil

1 pound boneless, skinless chicken breasts, cut into 1-inch-wide chunks

1 head broccoli, cut into florets (about 4 cups)

½ teaspoon freshly ground black pepper
½ teaspoon garlic powder or onion powder (salt-free)
Zest and juice of 1 lemon
2 tablespoons ground flaxseed
2 tablespoons reduced-sodium soy sauce
1 red or green bell pepper, chopped
1 small cucumber or zucchini, diced

Prepare the rice and set aside. Heat a large skillet over medium-high heat. Put in the olive oil, chicken, broccoli, black pepper, and garlic powder or onion powder. Cook 5 to 7 minutes, stirring often, until the chicken browns and is cooked through.

Turn the heat off and add the lemon zest and juice, flaxseed, and soy sauce. Toss to coat.

Divide the rice, bell pepper, and zucchini among four bowls and top with the chicken. Serve immediately.

Nutritional Stats Per serving (serving size: 3 cups) 369 calories, 32 g protein, 5 g sugars, 39 g carbohydrates, 9 g fat (1 g saturated), 72 mg cholesterol, 6 g fiber, 520 mg sodium

SALSA COD WITH GUACAMOLE

Cod is a mild-tasting fresh-water fish that is low in mercury and contains omega-3 fatty acids. It's primarily farmed, so search for U.S.-raised fish for the healthiest choice, since U.S. fish farms use closed recirculating systems.

Serves 4

Salsa Cod
Four 4-ounce cod fillets
½ cup jarred salsa
½ cup instant brown rice, cooked according to the package instructions

Guacamole
2 large ripe avocados, preferably Hass
1 ripe tomato, seeded and finely chopped (about 1 cup)
¼ cup red onion, minced
Juice of 2 limes (about ¼ cup)
1 jalapeño pepper, seeded and finely chopped (optional)
¼ cup minced fresh cilantro (optional)
¼ teaspoon sea salt

Preheat oven to 400°F. Place the fish in a 7 x 11-inch baking dish. Spread the salsa over the fish. Bake 15 to 18 minutes, until the fish flakes when pressed with a fork. Prepare the rice and set aside.

In the meantime, make the guacamole. Place the avocados, tomato, red onion, lime juice, jalapeño (if using), cilantro (if using), and salt in a large bowl. Use a wooden spoon to mash the ingredients together. Split into four even portions and serve immediately with the fish and rice.

Nutritional Stats Per serving (serving size: 1 piece cod with guacamole and rice) 413 calories, 27 g protein, 3 g sugars, 34 g carbohydrates, 20 g fat (3 g saturated), 57 mg cholesterol, 9 g fiber, 408 mg sodium

CHIPOTLE SALMON

Looking for a fast no-prep veggie fix to pour into your slow cooker? Add 2 cups of mixed frozen veggies to your cooker before you place the salmon fillets on top; there's no need to defrost.

Serves 4

    1 bunch asparagus, trimmed and cut into ⅓-inch pieces
    Zest and juice of 1 lime
    ¼ teaspoon salt
    2 tablespoons, chopped canned chipotle peppers in adobe sauce
    2 tablespoons no-salt-added tomato paste
    Four 4-ounce salmon fillets, skin on
    ¾ cup instant rice, cooked according to the package instructions

Place the asparagus in the slow cooker along with the lime zest and juice and salt. Toss well. Drizzle with 2 tablespoons water

Place the chipotle and tomato paste in a small bowl and mix well. Place the salmon, skin side down, on top of the asparagus and coat the tops of the fillets with the chipotle mixture. Cover and cook 2 to 2½ hours on low, until the salmon is still slightly pink in the center but no longer translucent. Serve immediately with the rice and asparagus.

Nutritional Stats Per serving (serving size: 1 piece salmon with ¼ pound asparagus and ⅓ cup rice) 397 calories, 29 g protein, 3 g sugars, 34 g carbohydrates, 16 g fat (4 g saturated), 62 mg cholesterol, 4 g fiber, 410 mg sodium

ITALIAN MEAT LOAF

Adding oats to your meat loaf might sound odd, but flavor-wise you won't notice the difference. Old-fashioned oats are a great swap for bread crumbs because the oats are fat-free and practically sodium-free, and give this healthier meat loaf the same tender texture as traditional recipes that use bread.

Serves 4

Meat Loaf

1 pound 90–93% lean ground beef

One 5-ounce package mushrooms or 2 cups chopped baby spinach

½ cup old-fashioned oats

¼ cup chopped parsley or basil (optional)

1 egg white

⅛ teaspoon freshly ground black pepper

OR raw meatball mixture from 1 recipe of Spaghetti and Meatballs (page 338)

½ cup low-sodium marinara sauce

Green Beans

2 teaspoons olive oil

1 pound green beans, trimmed and cut into thirds

1 lemon, cut in half

¼ cup chopped almonds

Place the ground beef, mushrooms or spinach, oats, parsley or basil, egg white, and black pepper in a large bowl. Mix well to combine, then form into a 4 x 8-inch loaf. Place in the center of a slow cooker and smooth the mixture with a spatula. Top with the marinara sauce and cook on high about 2 hours, until firm and cooked through.

While the meat loaf is cooking, make the green beans. Heat a large skillet over medium heat. Put in the olive oil and green beans. Cook 3 to 4 minutes, until the beans start to soften and brown. Reduce the heat to low and squeeze the lemon over the green beans. Sprinkle with the almonds and serve alongside the meat loaf.

Nutritional Stats Per serving (serving size: 2 large slices meat loaf, ½ pound green beans) 389 calories, 33 g protein, 7 g sugars, 29 g carbohydrates, 18 g fat (5 g saturated), 74 mg cholesterol, 8 g fiber, 338 mg sodium

20-DAY RECIPES: BLUE

Are you ready to get fully dialed in? If you're ready to tackle the blue level, then you probably made it through the yellow and orange levels without incident. The meals and snacks left you satisfied and the inches continued to melt away. But you can still tighten things up a bit by making a few more key swaps and by continuing to dial up the health on the awesome foods that you have always loved. You'll add more organic foods at this level, helping to further rid yourself of unwanted artificial ingredients and fillers. We'll also clean up your choices in other areas, like pasta, bread, and dairy.

SHOPPING LISTS: BLUE

This level will represent the healthiest choices you can make on this program. Having these foods at your disposal ensures that you are always reaching for body-friendly, health-packed foods that aren't weighted down with added sugars or unpronounceable chemicals.

WEEK 1

PRODUCE

3 pounds baby spinach or baby kale

One 12-ounce bunch curly kale

1 pound romaine lettuce

1 head butter lettuce

3 heads broccoli

1 head cabbage, such as savoy or napa

2 pounds green beans

2 bags carrots

2 bags celery stalks

1 tomato

One 5-ounce package mushrooms

4 red bell peppers

3 green bell peppers

1 jalapeño pepper

1 cucumber

3 large zucchini

1 small cucumber

3 red onions

3 yellow or white onions

4 heads garlic

3 avocados, preferably Hass

4 medium sweet potatoes

1 bunch fresh parsley

1 bunch cilantro

1 bunch fresh mint

11 apples, any variety

2 cups fresh berries, such as raspberries or blueberries

4 limes

2 lemons

1 pear

2 bananas

MEAT, POULTRY, AND FISH

1 pound 90–93% lean ground beef

2½ pounds ground turkey

2 pounds boneless, skinless chicken breasts

2½ pounds salmon fillets

1 pound cod fillets

1 pound medium peeled, deveined shrimp (about 22)

DAIRY

3 dozen eggs

½ gallon plain unsweetened coconut milk

¼ cup grated cheddar cheese or vegan cheese

2 cups shredded mozzarella cheese or vegan mozzarella

5 ounces feta cheese or vegan feta cheese

34 ounces plain, 2% Greek yogurt or coconut yogurt

½ cup grated Parmesan cheese or vegan grated cheese topping

One 8-ounce container sour cream or vegan sour cream

FROZEN

2 pounds frozen whole wheat or gluten-free pizza dough

One 8-ounce bag frozen mixed berries, such as raspberries, blueberries, or blackberries

GRAINS AND DRY GROCERIES

Four 9-inch gluten-free wraps (around 160 calories apiece)

8 slices whole wheat or gluten-free bread

8 hard corn taco shells or 8 small gluten-free soft tortillas

One 12-ounce bag quinoa

One 14-ounce box brown rice

½ cup seasoned whole wheat or gluten-free breadcrumbs

One 6-ounce bag lentils

1 cup old-fashioned oats

One 16-ounce bag chia seeds

One 5-ounce bag walnuts

One 5-ounce bag almonds

One 12-ounce container plant-based protein powder

OILS, CONDIMENTS, SPICES
One 25-ounce bottle olive oil
One 14-ounce jar coconut oil

JARRED AND CANNED GOODS
One 10-ounce jar pitted olives, such as kalamata
One 12-ounce container raisins
1 jar olive oil–based mayonnaise
Two 5-ounce cans tomato paste
Two 15-ounce cans no-salt-added diced tomatoes
Two 32-ounce containers low-sodium chicken or vegetable broth

4 ounces unsweetened, flaked coconut
16 bamboo skewers

One 5-ounce can cooking spray

Two 15-ounce cans low-sodium black beans
Two 15-ounce cans low-sodium beans, any variety
One 8-ounce can 100% pure pumpkin
One 12-ounce jar smooth peanut or almond butter
One 24-ounce jar low-sodium marinara sauce
One 15-ounce jar salsa

WEEK 2

PRODUCE
Two 10-ounce bunches kale
1 pound romaine lettuce leaves
8 ounces baby spinach
2 heads broccoli
1 pound green beans
1 bunch asparagus
Three 5-ounce packages mushrooms
4 tomatoes
4 green or red bell peppers
2 jalapeño peppers (optional)
3 cucumbers
2 bags carrots

1 bag celery stalks
7 onions, yellow or red
3 heads garlic
3 sweet potatoes
9 avocados, preferably Hass
1 bunch fresh mint
2 bunches fresh cilantro
1 bunch basil
8 apples
4 cups fresh berries, such as raspberries or blueberries
3 lemons
8 limes
1 pear

MEAT, POULTRY, AND FISH

1 pound cubed beef stew meat

2 pounds 90–93% lean ground beef

2½ pounds ground turkey

3 pounds boneless, skinless chicken breasts

2 pounds cod fillets

1 pound salmon fillets, skin on

DAIRY

2 dozen eggs

½ gallon plain, unsweetened coconut milk

1 cup crumbled feta cheese or vegan feta cheese

Three 5-ounce containers plain, 2% Greek yogurt or coconut yogurt

One 8-ounce container sour cream

½ cup grated Parmesan cheese or vegan grated cheese topping

8 ounces shredded mozzarella cheese or vegan mozzarella

FROZEN

1 pound frozen whole wheat or gluten-free pizza dough

8 ounces frozen blueberries

GRAINS AND DRY GROCERIES

One 26-ounce container whole-grain or gluten-free pancake mix

8 slices whole wheat, whole-grain gluten-free bread

4 small (6-inch) carb-control wraps or high-fiber gluten-free wraps

Four 9-inch gluten-free wraps (around 160 calories apiece)

16 hard corn taco shells or small gluten-free soft tortillas

One 14-ounce box instant brown rice

One 42-ounce container old-fashioned oats

One 12-ounce bag quinoa

One 4-ounce bar 70% cocoa

1 container stevia

One 5-ounce package walnuts

One 5-ounce package almonds

One 8-ounce bag bittersweet chocolate chips

OILS, CONDIMENTS, SPICES

One 5-ounce can cooking spray

JARRED AND CANNED GOODS

Three 15-ounce cans no-salt-added diced tomatoes

Four 5-ounce cans tomato paste

Two 24-ounce containers low-sodium chicken broth

Two 15-ounce cans low-sodium chickpeas

Two 15-ounce cans beans, any variety

One 15-ounce can low-sodium black beans

One 10-ounce jar black olives

One 24-ounce jar low-sodium marinara sauce

WEEK 3

PRODUCE

One 10-ounce bunch kale

2 pounds baby spinach

1 head broccoli

1 head butter lettuce

1 head cauliflower

1 head cabbage, such as napa or savoy

1 bunch asparagus

4 large sweet potatoes

20 ounces mushrooms, such as button or cremini

One 1-pound spaghetti squash

2 pounds green beans

2 bunches asparagus

4 red or green bell peppers

1 jalapeño pepper

1 tomato

2 zucchini

3 red or yellow onions

3 heads garlic

One 4-inch piece gingerroot

2 cups fresh berries, such as raspberries or blueberries

1 bunch fresh mint

2 bunches fresh parsley

2 bunches fresh cilantro

1 bunch fresh basil leaves

1 bunch scallions

4 avocados

4 apples, any variety

4 lemons

2 limes

1 pear

2 cups fresh berries, such as raspberries or blueberries

1 banana

1 lime

MEAT, POULTRY, AND FISH

4 pounds boneless, skinless chicken breasts

3 pounds 90–93% lean ground beef

3 pounds cod fillets

1/2 pound medium shrimp, shelled, deveined

DAIRY

3 dozen eggs

½ gallon plain, unsweetened coconut milk

One 15-ounce container part-skim ricotta cheese or tofu ricotta cheese

8 ounces shredded part-skim mozzarella cheese or vegan mozzarella

½ cup grated Parmesan cheese or vegan grated cheese topping

20 ounces plain, 2% Greek yogurt or coconut yogurt

8 ounces shredded cheddar cheese or vegan cheddar cheese

4 ounces feta cheese or vegan feta cheese

FROZEN

8 ounces frozen blueberries

1 pound frozen whole wheat or gluten-free pizza dough

GRAINS AND DRY GROCERIES

One 12-ounce box whole wheat or gluten-free lasagna noodles

4 small (6-inch) carb-control wraps or high-fiber gluten-free wraps

Two 8-inch whole wheat or gluten-free pitas (around 160 calories apiece)

8 small (6-inch) whole wheat or gluten-free tortillas

8 slices whole wheat or whole-grain gluten-free bread

6 ounces whole wheat or gluten-free spaghetti or angel hair pasta

One 26-ounce container whole-grain or gluten-free pancake mix

One 14-ounce box instant brown rice

One 5-ounce container almonds

One 5-ounce container walnuts

One 12-ounce package quinoa

1 container old-fashioned oats

One 12-ounce container chocolate plant-based protein powder

OILS, CONDIMENTS, SPICES

One 5-ounce can cooking spray

JARRED AND CANNED GOODS

One 28-ounce can diced tomatoes

Three 15-ounce cans chickpeas

Two 15-ounce cans black beans

One 15-ounce can low-sodium chicken or vegetable broth

One 15-ounce can low-sodium diced tomatoes

Two 24-ounce jars low-sodium marinara sauce

One 15-ounce jar salsa

One 10-ounce jar pitted olives, such as kalamata

20-DAY MEAL PLAN: BLUE

DAY 1

BREAKFAST

Pancakes

Chef's Note: You will save leftovers to make Tuesday's snack.

LUNCH

Chicken Fried Rice

Chef's Note: Be a conservationist! You'll use leftovers for lunch on Day 4.

SNACK

Sweet Potato Chips

Chef's Note: Don't overdo it on this snack. Use leftovers throughout the week.

DINNER

Spaghetti and Meatballs

Chef's Notes: Use leftover meatballs for lasagna and sub later in the week. Also use this time in the kitchen to prep Berry Delicious Yogurt Pops for the week.

DAY 2

BREAKFAST

Minty Lean and Green Shake

LUNCH

Italian Meat Loaf

SNACK

Trail Mix or Truffles

DINNER

Lasagna

Chef's Note: Use leftover meatballs from Day 1 to toss into this mix. And use this time to make sweet potatoes in the slow cooker for Sweet Potato Soup and Sweet Potato Skins later on.

DAY 3

BREAKFAST

Scrambles to Go

LUNCH

Meatball Sub

SNACK

Spiced Chickpeas and Nuts

DINNER

Shrimp Scampi

DESSERT

Berry Delicious Frozen Yogurt Pops

DAY 4

BREAKFAST

Baked Apple Parfait

Chef's Note: Use leftover apples from the previous week, if possible.

LUNCH

Chicken Fried Rice

Chef's Note: Time-saver! This is leftover from earlier in the week.

SNACK

Sweet Potato Skins

Chef's Note: These will be made from leftover slow-cooker sweet potatoes from Day 1.

DINNER

Salsa Cod with Guacamole

Chef's Note: Be sure to save the leftover guacamole for the snack on Thursday. Also, during this time, defrost the pizza dough to make empanadas tomorrow.

DAY 5

BREAKFAST

Cinnamon Nut Breakfast Cereal

LUNCH

Empanadas

SNACK

Chocolate Peanut Butter Banana Protein Shake

DINNER

Shrimp Scampi

Chef's Note: Get the most out of this prep time by storing leftovers for shrimp cocktail snack tomorrow.

DAY 6

BREAKFAST

Zesty Breakfast Taco

LUNCH
Empanadas

SNACK
Shrimp Cocktail

DINNER
Baked Pesto Cod or Chipotle Salmon

Chef's Notes: The tasty cod can be used again tomorrow! Save the leftovers for Cod Tacos on Day 7.

DAY 7

BREAKFAST
French Toast

LUNCH
Cod Tacos

SNACK
Afternoon Wake-Up Call

DINNER
Slow Cooker Chicken Enchilada

DESSERT
No-Bake Peanut Butter Coconut Truffles

DAY 8

BREAKFAST
Pancakes

Chef's Note: You will save leftovers to make Day 10's snack.

LUNCH
Chicken Fried Rice

Chef's Note: Be a conservationist! You'll use leftovers for lunch on Day 11.

SNACK

Sweet Potato Chips

Chef's Note: Don't overdo it on this snack. Use leftovers throughout the week.

DINNER

Spaghetti and Meatballs

Chef's Note: Use leftover meatballs for lasagna and sub later in the week. Also use this time in the kitchen to prep Berry Delicious Yogurt Pops for the week.

DAY 9

BREAKFAST

Minty Lean and Green Shake

LUNCH

Italian Meat Loaf

SNACK

Trail Mix or Truffles

DINNER

Lasagna

Chef's Note: Use leftover meatballs from Day 8 to toss into this mix. And use this time to make sweet potatoes in the slow cooker for Sweet Potato Soup and Sweet Potato Skins later on.

DAY 10

BREAKFAST

Scrambles to Go

LUNCH

Meatball Sub

SNACK
Spiced Chickpeas and Nuts

DINNER
Shrimp Scampi

DESSERT
Berry Delicious Yogurt Pops

DAY 11

BREAKFAST
Baked Apple Parfait

Chef's Note: Use leftover slow cooker apples from the previous week, if possible.

LUNCH
Chicken Fried Rice

Chef's Note: Time-saver! This is leftover from earlier in the week.

SNACK
Sweet Potato Skins

Chef's Note: These will be made from leftover slow cooker sweet potatoes from Day 8.

DINNER
Salsa Cod with Guacamole

Chef's Note: Be sure to save the leftover guacamole for the snack on Day 12. Also, during this time, defrost the pizza dough to make empanadas tomorrow.

DAY 12

BREAKFAST
Cinnamon Nut Breakfast Cereal

LUNCH
Empanadas

SNACK

Chocolate Peanut Butter Banana
Protein Shake

DINNER

Shrimp Scampi

Chef's Note: Get the most out
of this prep time by storing
leftovers for shrimp cocktail snack
tomorrow.

DAY 13

BREAKFAST

Zesty Breakfast Taco

LUNCH

Empanadas

SNACK

Shrimp Cocktail

DINNER

Baked Pesto Cod or Chipotle
Salmon

Chef's Note: This tasty cod can be
used again tomorrow! Save the
leftovers for Cod Tacos on Day 14.

DAY 14

BREAKFAST

French Toast

LUNCH

Cod Tacos

SNACK

Afternoon Wake-Up Call

DINNER

Slow Cooker Chicken Enchilada

DESSERT

No-Cook Chia Pudding

DAY 15

BREAKFAST

Pancakes

Chef's Note: You will save leftovers to make Day 17's snack.

LUNCH

Chicken Fried Rice

Chef's Note: Be a conservationist! You'll use leftovers for lunch on Day 18.

SNACK

Sweet Potato Chips

Chef's Note: Don't overdo it on this snack. Use leftovers throughout the week.

DINNER

Spaghetti and Meatballs

Chef's Note: Use leftover meatballs for lasagna and sub later in the week. Also use this time in the kitchen to prep Berry Delicious Yogurt Pops for the week.

DAY 16

BREAKFAST

Minty Lean and Green Shake

LUNCH

Italian Meat Loaf

SNACK

Trail Mix

DINNER

Lasagna

Chef's Note: Use leftover meatballs from Day 15 to toss into this mix. And use this time to make sweet potatoes in the slow cooker for Sweet Potato Soup and Sweet Potato Skins later on.

DAY 17

BREAKFAST

Scrambles to Go

LUNCH

Meatball Sub

SNACK

Spiced Chickpeas and Nuts

DINNER

Shrimp Scampi

DESSERT

Berry Delicious Yogurt Pops

DAY 18

BREAKFAST

Baked Apple Parfait

Chef's Note: Use leftover slow cooker apples from the previous week, if possible.

LUNCH

Chicken Fried Rice

Chef's Note: Time-saver! This is leftover from earlier in the week.

SNACK

Sweet Potato Skins

Chef's Note: These will be made from leftover slow-cooker sweet potatoes from Day 15.

DINNER

Salsa Cod with Guacamole

Chef's Note: Be sure to save the leftover guacamole for the snack on Thursday. Also, during this time, defrost the pizza dough to make empanadas tomorrow.

DAY 19

BREAKFAST

Cinnamon Nut Breakfast Cereal

LUNCH

Empanadas

SNACK

Chocolate Peanut Butter Banana Protein Shake

DINNER

Shrimp Scampi

Chef's Note: Get the most out of this prep time by storing leftovers for shrimp cocktail snack tomorrow.

DAY 20

BREAKFAST

Zesty Breakfast Taco

LUNCH

Empanadas

SNACK

Shrimp Cocktail

DINNER

Baked Pesto Cod or Chipotle Salmon

Chef's Note: This tasty dish can be used again tomorrow!

20-DAY RECIPES: BLUE

Now you really get to test your kitchen muscle. What have you learned in the first 20-day programs about food preparation and healthier choices that is going to make these 20 days a cinch? Chances are you have perfected your time management and meal prep in the kitchen so these next 20 days will be a breeze. These recipes make great meals and snacks that you can serve yourself, your family, or your friends, completely guilt-free.

BREAKFASTS

PANCAKES

Chia seeds aren't just for sprouting pottery pets: they can power your day with high levels of protein, fiber, and good-quality fats like omega-3s. Shop for them in health food stores or buy in bulk online and have them delivered straight to your door.

Serves 4, makes twelve 3-inch pancakes

¾ cup whole-grain or gluten-free pancake mix
⅓ cup protein powder
2 tablespoons ground flaxseed or chia seeds
¾ cup plain, unsweetened coconut milk
1 egg
2 teaspoons lemon zest (from 1 medium lemon), optional
Cooking spray
1 cup fresh berries, such as raspberries or blueberries

Place the pancake mix, protein powder, and flaxseed or chia seeds in a large bowl. Mix well with a whisk. Add the coconut milk, egg, and lemon zest if using. Whisk well until just combined.

Coat a large skillet with cooking spray. Set over medium heat. Using a ¼-cup scoop, ladle out four scoops of batter, 1 inch apart. Cook 2 to 3 minutes, until bubbles start to form around the edges.

Flip and cook 2 to 3 minutes more, until the pancakes are cooked through. Transfer to a plate and repeat with remaining batter. Sprinkle with the berries and serve immediately.

Choosing chia? Then your pancakes will remind you of those sinful coffee shop lemon poppy seed muffins. Enjoy the same zesty zing of lemon without hundreds of extra calories hiding in those buttery muffin tops.

Nutritional Stats Per serving (serving size: 3 pancakes plus berries) 204 calories, 8 g protein, 3 g sugars, 34 g carbohydrates, 4 g fat (1 g saturated), 46 mg cholesterol, 4 g fiber (fiber went down because we did gluten-free mix), 269 mg sodium

Chef's Notes: You can use the same batter to make waffles. Add 2 tablespoons chopped nuts, like walnuts, to add crunch and protein to the batter. Also, with gluten-free pancake mixes you don't need to worry about overmixing since there is no gluten to make the pancakes tough.

MINTY LEAN AND GREEN SHAKE

Swapping out sugar for stevia will kick your fat-burning ability into higher gear since sugar raises blood sugar, making it easier for your body to store fat. If you're missing the sweet taste of sugar, try adding a little vanilla extract to tempt your palate the sugar-free way.

Serves 2

1 cup kale
3 stalks celery
½ ripe pear, seeded
2 scoops protein powder (about ⅔ cup)
1½ cups plain, unsweetened coconut milk
2 tablespoons fresh mint
1 tablespoon chia seeds
1 tablespoon stevia
½ teaspoon vanilla extract (optional)
8 ice cubes

Place all the ingredients in a blender along with ½ cup water and blend until very smooth. Serve immediately.

Nutritional Stats Per serving (serving size: 1½ cups) 250 calories, 20 g protein, 28 grams sugars, 28 g carbohydrates, 8 g fat (5 g saturated), 0 mg cholesterol, 7 g fiber, 177 mg sodium

SCRAMBLES TO GO

Carb-control wraps are soft and tasty, just like all white flour wraps. They're an easy way to bump up fiber, which feeds good bacteria cultures in your digestive system and helps you absorb vitamins and and burn fat more efficiently.

Serves 4

Cooking spray
3 cups chopped mushrooms, asparagus, or spinach
6 eggs
4 egg whites or ½ cup egg whites from the carton
4 small (6-inch) carb-control wraps or high-fiber gluten-free wraps, cut in half

Coat a large skillet with cooking spray. Set over high heat and add the mushrooms, asparagus, or spinach. Cook 2 to 3 minutes, stirring often, until the vegetable softens. Lower the heat to medium and carefully add another layer of the cooking spray.

Add the eggs and cook 3 to 4 minutes more, scrambling the egg mixture continuously with a fork or spatula, until soft curds form.

Divide the egg between the wrap halves and serve immediately or cover in aluminum foil to go.

Nutritional Stats Per serving (serving size: 1 small wrap stuffed with eggs) 327 calories, 17 g protein, 2 g sugars, 36 g carbohydrates, 12 g fat (3 g saturated), 279 mg cholesterol, 5 g fiber, 503 mg sodium

BAKED APPLE BREAKFAST PARFAIT

Don't restrict your protein powder to shakes alone. Sneaking protein into other recipes makes them more filling and is a clever way for vegetarians to build more protein into their meals.

Serves 4

8 baked apple halves
1½ cups plain, 2% Greek yogurt or coconut yogurt
⅓ cup protein powder
2 teaspoons stevia

Cut each baked apple half into 4 even strips. Place the yogurt in a small bowl along with the protein powder, stevia, and 2 tablespoons water. Stir well

Layer ¼ cup of the yogurt mixture into 4 glasses, top each with 2 slices of the apple, repeat with the remaining yogurt and apple slices, and serve.

Nutritional Stats Per serving (serving size: 1 parfait) 318 calories, 14 g protein, 32 g sugars, 40 g carbohydrates, 14 g fat (3 g saturated), 6 mg cholesterol, 6 g fiber, 49 mg sodium

CINNAMON NUT BREAKFAST CEREAL

Out of berries? Add 1 cup thinly sliced, high-fiber pear and a drizzle of almond extract for a flavor swap. Pears are not only high in fiber but also high in copper, an essential mineral that is required to manufacture collagen.

Serves 4

1 cup old-fashioned oats
½ cup quinoa, rinsed under cold running water if not prewashed (see Chef's Tip)
4 scoops protein powder (1⅓ cups)
1 teaspoon cinnamon
¼ cup chopped nuts, such as walnuts or almonds
2 teaspoons stevia
1 cup fresh berries, such as raspberries or blueberries

Place the oats, quinoa, protein powder, and cinnamon in a medium saucepan. Add 6½ cups of water and bring to a simmer over medium-low heat. Cover and cook 10 to 15 minutes, stirring often, until the quinoa is tender. Top with nuts and berries. Serve immediately.

Nutritional Stats Per serving (serving size: 2 cups) 319 calories, 26 g protein, 4 g sugars, 38 g carbohydrates, 10 g fat (2 g saturated), 0 mg cholesterol, 9 g fiber, 82 mg sodium

Chef's Note: Don't wash your berries until just before you use them, as washing can damage their delicate skins and cause quicker spoilage..

ZESTY BREAKFAST TACO

Adding antioxidant-rich foods like beans provides a lot more than just energy. Black beans in particular, more than other types of beans or even lentils, have special insoluble fibers that clean your colon, the lower part of our digestive tract that usually doesn't get the attention it needs.

Serves 4

4 eggs
4 egg whites or ½ cup egg whites from the carton
¼ cup jarred salsa or pesto (page 265 or page 342)
Cooking spray
2 cups baby spinach
½ cup canned black beans, drained and rinsed
8 small (6-inch) whole wheat or gluten-free tortillas

Place the eggs, egg whites, and salsa or pesto in a medium bowl. Gently whisk to combine.

Coat a large skillet with cooking spray and place it over high heat. Add the spinach and cook 1 to 2 minutes, turning often, until wilted. Stir in the beans. Transfer to a plate and set aside.

Coat the same large skillet with more cooking spray. Add the eggs and cook 2 to 3 minutes, scrambling them with a fork as they cook. Add the cooked spinach and beans.

Set out the tortillas. Scoop a quarter of the eggs onto each tortilla and fold the tortilla over to form a taco. Serve immediately.

Nutritional Stats Per serving (serving size: 2 filled tacos) 257 calories, 16 g protein, 1 g sugars, 33 g carbohydrates, 9 g fat (3 g saturated), 186 mg cholesterol, 6 g fiber, 573 mg sodium

FRENCH TOAST

Most gluten-free breads, wraps, and bread mixers tend to be much lower in fiber compared with whole wheat or whole-grain versions. To remedy this, add in naturally gluten-free ground flaxseed, chia seeds, or canned pumpkin, ¼ cup per recipe. Also, shop for gluten-free bread made with 100 percent whole grains like quinoa, amaranth, and buckwheat.

Serves 4

1 cup plain, unsweetened coconut milk
1 egg
2 egg whites
⅓ cup protein powder
1 teaspoon vanilla extract
¼ teaspoon ground cinnamon
8 slices whole-grain or gluten-free bread
2 tablespoons chia seeds
Cooking spray
1 cup fresh berries, such as raspberries or blueberries

Place the coconut milk, egg, egg white, protein powder, vanilla, and cinnamon in a large, shallow dish and whisk well. Using the tines of a fork, poke the bread several times to allow better absorption of the liquid. Transfer the bread slices to a tray and sprinkle with the chia seeds.

Coat a large skillet with cooking spray and place it over medium heat. Dip four of the bread slices into the egg mixture and transfer to the skillet. Cook 2 to 3 minutes per side until golden, then turn. Cook 2 to 3 minutes more, until a crisp crust has formed. Transfer to a plate and repeat with cooking spray and remaining bread. Top with berries and serve immediately.

Nutritional Stats Per serving (serving size: 2 slices French toast, ¼ cup berries) 309 calories, 17 g protein, 12 g sugars, 48 g carbohydrates, 5 g fat (2 g saturated), 46 mg cholesterol, 10 g fiber, 457 mg sodium

SNACKS

SWEET POTATO CHIPS

If you're looking for a salt-free version of this recipe, simply top your chips with any ground spice from cumin to chili powder, or use homemade Chef Rocco's Seasoning Salt without the salt (page 344).

Serves 4

4 large sweet potatoes, skin on
1 tablespoon olive oil
½ teaspoon Old Bay or Chef Rocco's Seasoning Salt

Preheat oven to 400°F. Wash the sweet potatoes under cold running water: do not peel, dry well with a dishtowel. Using a vegetable slicer (page 113) or Japanese mandolin, cut the potatoes into ⅛-inch slices. Transfer to a large bowl along with the olive oil and seasoning salt, and toss well. Spread the chips out on ungreased baking sheets and bake 8 to 10 minutes, until they are crisp and start to brown. Transfer to a plate and serve immediately.

Nutritional Stats Per serving (serving size: 15 to 20 chips) 153 calories, 2 g protein, 6 g sugars, 29 g carbohydrates, 3 g fat (0 g saturated), 0 mg cholesterol, 4 g fiber, 127 mg sodium

TRAIL MIX

The nutritional stats of most store-bought trail mixes resemble bagged candies. One cup can clock in at over 500 calories with more than 40 grams of sugar.

Serves 8

One 15-ounce can chickpeas, drained and well rinsed
¾ cup old-fashioned oats
¼ cup chopped nuts, such as walnuts or almonds
3 tablespoons chia seeds
3 tablespoons protein powder
2 egg whites
¼ teaspoon seasoning salt
Cooking spray
⅓ cup raisins

Preheat oven to 400°F. In a large bowl, combine the chickpeas, oats, nuts, chia seeds, protein powder, egg whites, and seasoning salt.

Cover a large baking sheet with aluminum foil and coat with cooking spray. Spread the chickpea mixture out over the foil and bake 12 to 15 minutes, stirring once or twice during baking, until golden. Remove the baking sheet from the oven and sprinkle with the raisins. Let cool on the sheet 5 to 6 minutes, then serve. Or let cool completely and store in ziplock bags on the countertop for up to 5 days.

Nutritional Stats Per serving (serving size: ¾ cup trail mix) 178 calories, 9 g protein, 8 g sugars, 25 g carbohydrates, 6 g fat (1 g saturated), 0 mg cholesterol, 6 g fiber, 182 mg sodium

NO-BAKE PEANUT BUTTER COCONUT TRUFFLES

Learn how to tame your sweet tooth. Yes, it can be done! When you gradually lower your sugar intake, your taste for sweets will diminish and you'll be happier with less and won't miss overly sugary treats that you used to eat.

Serves 5, makes 10 truffles

    1 scoop protein powder, vanilla, chocolate, or peanut butter flavor (⅓ cup)
    2 tablespoons natural peanut butter
    2 tablespoons unsweetened, shredded coconut, plus 1 additional tablespoon
        (or 1 tablespoon unsweetened cocoa powder) for rolling
    1 teaspoon honey
    1 tablespoon coconut oil
    1 teaspoon cinnamon

Place the protein powder, peanut butter, 2 tablespoons shredded coconut, honey, coconut oil, and cinnamon into a small bowl and mash with the back of a spoon until a thick, dry paste starts to form.

Start to mix together, adding a few drops of water at a time, until the mixture starts to clump and becomes sticky. Using your hands, roll into 10 small (½-inch diameter) balls. Roll into the additional coconut or cocoa powder. Store in an airtight container in the refrigerator for up to 3 days or consume immediately.

Nutritional Stats Per serving (serving size: 2 truffles) 97 calories, 5 g protein, 2 g sugars, 4 g carbohydrates, 7 g fat (4 g saturated), 0 mg cholesterol, 1 g fiber, 46 mg sodium

SPICED CHICKPEAS AND NUTS

Making your own snacks means you can build them with nutrient-dense superfoods like beans. Most packaged chips offer little in the way of nutrition and pump you up with empty carb calories that can't satisfy because they don't come with protein or fiber the way beans do.

Serves 6

Two 15-ounce cans low-sodium chickpeas, drained and well rinsed
3 tablespoons olive oil
½ teaspoon cumin
½ teaspoon chili powder
½ teaspoon ginger
¼ teaspoon cayenne pepper
1 cup chopped walnuts

Preheat the oven to 400°F. Drain and rinse the chickpeas and lay them out on paper towels, rubbing gently to dry.

Transfer the chickpeas to a large bowl along with the olive oil and the spices. Toss well and transfer to a rimmed baking sheet, lined with aluminum foil.

Bake for 30 to 35 minutes, until the chickpeas start to brown. Add the nuts and stir well. Bake 5 additional minutes, until the nuts start to brown and the chickpeas are crisp. Serve warm, or let cool completely and store on the countertop in an airtight container for up to 5 days.

Nutritional Stats Per serving (serving size: ¾ cup) 167 calories, 7 g protein, 7 g sugars, 19 g carbohydrates, 7 g fat (1 g saturated), 0 mg cholesterol, 6 g fiber, 244 mg sodium

SWEET POTATO SKINS

An entertaining-worthy meal that's on your *20-Minute Body* plan, perfect for game time, movie night, or even an impromptu night in with the girls. Let your slow cooker do the work, while you catch up on your workout, or catch up on a few errands, or make your home party-ready.

Serves 4

2 tablespoons olive oil–based mayonnaise
1 tablespoon minced chipotle peppers in adobo sauce

2 large sweet potatoes or yams, cut in half
4 tablespoons salsa, mild or hot
2 scallions, thinly sliced, or ¼ cup minced red onion

Mix the mayonnaise and the chipotle in a small bowl, and set aside. Place the potato halves, skin side down, in the slow cooker. Spread 1 tablespoon of the salsa over each potato half and start the slow cooker at high. Cook 2 to 2½ hours, until the potatoes are fork-tender, but the skins are still intact.

Remove the potatoes and scoop out the flesh, leaving a ¼-inch rim inside each potato. Transfer the flesh to a large bowl and mix in the scallions or onion. Cut each of the halved potato shells halves into 4 pieces and transfer to a baking sheet lined with aluminum foil. Divide the filling among the sliced potato shells and place under the broiler for 2 to 3 minutes, until the tops brown. Remove, drizzle with the chipotle mayo, and serve.

Nutritional Stats Per serving (serving size: 4 filled sweet potato skins) 155 calories, 3 g protein, 7 g sugars, 31 g carbohydrates, 3 g fat (0 g saturated), 3 mg cholesterol, 5 g fiber, 330 mg sodium

CHOCOLATE PEANUT BUTTER BANANA PROTEIN SHAKE

This is a great recipe that you can modify by trying different protein powder flavors, adding frozen berries or bananas, or using PB2 instead of full-fat peanut butter. Since it is ice blended, this shake keeps well as a snack at work if you make it in the morning.

Serves 2

1 scoop chocolate protein powder
1 cup coconut milk
½ ripe banana
1 tablespoon natural peanut butter
8 ice cubes
¼ teaspoon cinnamon

Combine all ingredients in a blender and blend until smooth. Add ½ to ¾ cup of water for a thinner shake. Serve immediately or store in an airtight drink bottle to take to school or your office.

Nutritional Stats Per serving (serving size: 1 shake, about 1½ cups) 166 calories, 15 g protein, 12 g sugars, 18 g carbohydrates, 5 g fat (1 g saturated), 3 mg cholesterol, 3 g fiber, 129 mg sodium

SHRIMP COCKTAIL BITES

Want to create a healthy cocktail party but not sure what to serve? Before your guests arrive, whip up a few easy appetizer platters with ingredients you already have on hand. Start with these savory bites, chipotle deviled eggs (page 248), and spicy peanut avocado pancakes (page 292).

Serves 4

½ pound medium shrimp, shelled, deveined, and chopped
½ teaspoon chili powder
OR ¼ pound leftover shrimp from Baked Shrimp Scampi (page 340)
1 zucchini, cubed (about 2 cups)
1 tablespoon olive oil
8 butter lettuce leaves
4 teaspoons cocktail sauce

Place the shrimp and chili powder in a bowl with the zucchini and toss well. Heat a large skillet over medium-high heat. Put in the olive oil and the shrimp/zucchini mixture and cook 3 to 4 minutes, stirring often, until the shrimp have turned pink and are no longer translucent in the center and the zucchini is soft.

Set out the 8 butter lettuce leaves and place ½ teaspoon of the cocktail sauce on each leaf. Divide the shrimp mixture among them. Serve immediately.

Nutritional Stats Per serving (serving size: 2 lettuce leaves with ¼ cup shrimp mixture) 115 calories, 9 g protein, 3 g sugars, 4 g carbohydrates, 8 g fat (1 g saturated), 71 mg cholesterol, 1 g fiber, 381 mg sodium

AFTERNOON WAKE-UP CALL

Blueberries are great when it comes to antioxidant load, and they may also be able to improve your work performance since studies say they are natural memory boosters!

Serves 2

1½ cups blueberries
1 scoop protein powder (⅓ cup)
1 cup plain, unsweetened coconut
1 cup packed baby spinach
½ ripe avocado (about ½ cup flesh)
2 teaspoons stevia

Place all the ingredients in a mini chopper, Magic Bullet, or Ninja blender along with 1 cup of water (adjust for desired thickness). Blend until smooth and serve.

Nutritional Stats Per serving (serving size: 1 shake, about 2 cups) 220 calories, 12 g protein, 11 g sugars, 24 g carbohydrates, 10 g fat (4 g saturated), 0 mg cholesterol, 7 g fiber, 93 mg sodium

LUNCHES

CHICKEN FRIED RICE

Looking to dabble with a gluten-free lifestyle? Then do it the healthiest way possible and ditch high-sugar, highly processed packaged foods that are gluten-free but still aren't very good for you. To stock your pantry with a few healthier items, look for naturally salt- and sugar-free whole grains like brown rice, quinoa, and gluten-free oats.

Serves 4

1 cup instant brown rice

1 tablespoon olive oil

2 boneless, skinless chicken breasts, cut into ¼-inch thin strips

5 cups assorted chopped veggies, such as asparagus, mushrooms, and bell peppers

2 garlic cloves, minced

One 1-inch piece gingerroot, minced

2 tablespoons balsamic vinegar

1 tablespoon hot sauce (optional)

¼ teaspoon salt

1 egg

Cook the brown rice according to the package instructions and set aside. Heat a large skillet over medium heat. Put in the olive oil, then the chicken and the vegetables at once, and increase the heat to high. Cook 3 to 4 minutes, stirring often, until the chicken and vegetables begin to brown. Add the garlic and the ginger and cook 1 minute more, until they become fragrant.

Reduce the heat to medium and add the rice, vinegar, hot sauce if using, and salt. Add the egg and cook an additional 2 minutes, stirring often, until the vegetables are well incorporated with the rice and the egg is cooked through. Serve immediately.

Nutritional Stats Per serving (serving size: 2 cups) 357 calories, 25 g protein, 5 g sugars, 45 g carbohydrates, 8 g fat (2 g saturated), 101 mg cholesterol, 4 g fiber, 270 mg sodium

ITALIAN MEAT LOAF

Like old-fashioned oats, cooked quinoa works well in meat mixtures, breakfast foods like pancakes and eggs, and even desserts as long as you cook it first. This meat loaf is an iron source, giving you more than 30 percent of your daily needs per serving and containing both heme and nonheme iron.

Serves 4

Meat Loaf
1 pound 90–93% lean ground beef
One 5-ounce package mushrooms, or 2 cups chopped baby spinach
½ cup quinoa, cooked according to package directions
¼ cup chopped parsley or basil (optional)
1 egg white
¼ teaspoon salt
⅛ teaspoon freshly ground black pepper
OR raw meatball mixture from 1 recipe of Spaghetti and Meatballs (page 338)
½ cup low-sodium marinara sauce

Green Beans
Cooking spray
1 pound green beans, trimmed and cut crosswise into thirds
1 lemon, cut in half
¼ cup chopped almonds

Place the beef, mushrooms or spinach, quinoa, parsley or basil, egg white, salt, and black pepper in a large bowl. Mix well to combine, then form into a 4 x 8-inch loaf. Place in the center of a slow cooker and smooth the mixture with a spatula. Top with the marinara sauce, and cook on high about 2 hours, until firm and cooked through.

While the meat loaf is cooking, make the green beans. Coat a large skillet with cooking spray and place it over medium heat. Add the green beans. Cook 3 to 4 minutes, until the beans start to soften and brown. Reduce the heat to low and squeeze the lemon over the green beans. Sprinkle with the almonds and serve alongside the meat loaf.

Nutritional Stats Per serving (serving size: 2 large slices meat loaf, ¼ pound green beans) 350 calories, 30 g protein, 6 g sugars, 21 g carbohydrates, 17 g fat (5 g saturated), 74 mg cholesterol, 7 g fiber, 338 mg sodium

MEATBALL SUB

As you go through the phases from yellow to blue you'll also learn to adjust the portion size of certain foods, especially those that are high-salt and high-carb. The great news is that high-intensity superfoods like spinach, kale, and broccoli will take their place so you'll still get the same portion with superior nutrition and less calories.

Serves 4

1 pound 90–93% lean ground beef
One 5-ounce package mushrooms, finely chopped
½ cup grated Parmesan or vegan grated cheese topping cheese
¼ cup chopped parsley or basil (optional)
1 egg white
⅛ teaspoon freshly ground black pepper
1 tablespoon olive oil (optional)
2 cups low-sodium marinara sauce
2 cups baby spinach leaves
Two 8-inch whole wheat pitas (around 160 calories apiece), or gluten-free pitas, cut in half

Place the beef, mushrooms, Parmesan, parsley or basil if using, egg white, and black pepper in a large bowl. Mix well and form into 12 meatballs, 2 inches in diameter (about 2 tablespoons raw meat mixture).

Transfer to a slow cooker, top with the marinara sauce, and cook 1½ hours on low. Or use leftover meatballs from Spaghetti and Meatballs (page 338), without the pasta.

To assemble the subs, tuck a few baby spinach leaves into each pita half. Put three meatballs on top of the spinach and serve immediately or wrap with aluminum foil and refrigerate up to 5 hours before serving.

Nutritional Stats Per serving (serving size: ½ large whole wheat pita with 3 meatballs) 392 calories, 35 g protein, 8 g sugars, 28 g carbohydrates, 15 g fat (6 g saturated), 82 mg cholesterol, 3 g fiber, 658 mg sodium

EMPANADAS

Empanadas can be made with a variety of fillings! If you have leftover Turkey Chili (page 301), drain the broth and use it for zesty turkey empanadas in place of the filling below.

Serves 4

    1 tablespoon olive oil
    1 head broccoli, cut into small florets (about 4 cups)
    ½ red onion, thinly sliced
    ¼ cup pitted olives, such as kalamata
    2 tablespoons raisins
    1 teaspoon dried herbs, such as thyme
    1 pound whole wheat or gluten-free pizza dough, defrosted and cut into quarters
    ¼ cup grated cheddar cheese or vegan cheese

Preheat oven to 400°F. Place a large skillet over medium heat. Put in the olive oil, broccoli, onion, olives, raisins, and dried herbs. Cook 3 to 4 minutes, stirring occasionally, until the broccoli starts to brown and soften. Reduce the heat to low and add a few tablespoons of water. Cover and cook 1 minute more, until the broccoli is tender. Turn off the heat and let cool while you prepare the dough.

Roll the dough out into 4-inch-diameter disks, or stretch the dough out with your hands. Set out a large baking sheet and place the disks a few inches apart. Place 1 tablespoon of the cheese on each disk. Divide the broccoli mixture among the four disks and pinch–fold over one edge to make a half-moon shape. Pinch the edges shut with your fingers and bake 10 to 12 minutes, until the dough is cooked through and brown around the edges. Let cool 5 minutes before serving.

Nutritional Stats Per serving (serving size: 1 large empanada) 355 calories, 13 g protein, 12 g sugars, 62 g carbohydrates, 7 g fat (2 g saturated), 7 mg cholesterol, 7 g fiber, 611 mg sodium

COD TACOS

Have a few broken taco shells at the bottom of the box? Don't toss them! Place fish and broken taco shells over crisp romaine lettuce for a satisfying taco salad.

Serves 4

    2 cups baby spinach
    2 cups cilantro leaves

2 tablespoons olive oil
⅛ teaspoon salt
Four 4-ounce cod fillets
OR leftover baked cod (page 342)
2 cups thinly sliced napa or savoy cabbage
Juice of 1 lime
8 hard corn taco shells or 8 small gluten-free soft tortillas

Preheat oven to 400°F. To make the pesto, place the spinach, cilantro, olive oil, and salt in a food processor. Process until a chunky mixture forms. Divide the pesto into four portions and spread over each piece of fish in a baking dish. Bake 18 to 20 minutes, until the fish flakes when pressed with a fork.

Combine the cabbage and lime juice, and toss well. Break the cooked cod into pieces. Layer half a cod fillet in each taco shell, with ¼ cup of the cabbage mixture. Serve immediately.

Nutritional Stats Per serving (serving size: 2 tacos with ½ cup cabbage) 330 calories, 27 g protein, 0 g sugars, 20 g carbohydrates, 17 g fat (4 g saturated), 65 mg cholesterol, 3 g fiber, 435 mg sodium

DINNERS

SPAGHETTI AND MEATBALLS

Spaghetti squash at only 42 calories a cup is an incredibly low-cal sub for pasta! Simply steam it and shred with a fork; it naturally forms firm noodle-like shreds. Let leftover squash cool completely before storing it in an airtight container to reheat later for fast, lower-carb meals compared with white pasta.

Serves 4

1 pound 90–93% lean ground beef
One 5-ounce package mushrooms
¼ cup chopped parsley or basil (optional)
1 egg
¼ teaspoon salt
⅛ teaspoon freshly ground black pepper
One 28-ounce can diced tomatoes
One 1-pound spaghetti squash

Place the beef, mushrooms, parsley or basil if using, egg, salt, and black pepper in a bowl. Mix well and form into twelve 2-inch-diameter meatballs, (about 2 tablespoon raw meat mixture). Transfer to a slow cooker, top with the canned diced tomatoes, and cook 1½ hours on low.

To cook the squash: Bring 2 inches of water to a boil in a large stockpot. Add the squash, cover, and allow to steam for 7 to 10 minutes, adjusting the level of water as needed. Allow squash to cool for 5 minutes. When cool, shred the squash with a fork.

Serve the meatballs over the spaghetti squash.

Nutritional Stats Per serving (serving size: 3 meatballs with ¼ pound spaghetti squash) 305 calories, 28 g protein, 8 g sugars, 17 g carbohydrates, 13 g fat (5 g saturated), 120 mg cholesterol, 4 g fiber, 553 mg sodium

LASAGNA

Looking to take your lasagna over the top with taste without increasing calories? Shop for fresh whole wheat or gluten-free lasagna noodles instead of the dry noodles that are much tougher.

Serves 8

Filling
One 15-ounce container part-skim ricotta cheese or tofu ricotta cheese
4 cups chopped baby spinach
1 zucchini, grated
1 egg
3 cups low-sodium marinara sauce
OR cooked meatballs with tomatoes, from Spaghetti and Meatballs (page 338)
One 12-ounce box whole wheat or gluten-free lasagna noodles
2 cups grated part-skim mozzarella cheese or vegan mozzarella cheese

If using ricotta filling, place the ricotta, spinach, zucchini, and egg in a large bowl and stir well. Spread out half the marinara sauce into a 13 x 9-inch baking dish. Cook the lasagna noodles for 5 to 6 minutes and drain. Cover the sauce with a layer of lasagna noodles. Top with half the ricotta mixture and then with more lasagna noodles. Top with the remaining ricotta and with the remaining noodles. Top with remaining marinara and sprinkle with the mozzarella. Bake 45 to 50 minutes, uncovered, until the cheese has melted and the edges are lightly browned. Let cool 5 minutes before cutting into eight squares and serving.

If using meatballs, cut each meatball in half. Cook the lasagna noodles for 5 to 6 minutes and drain. Spread out half the diced tomatoes with their juices into a 13 x 9-inch baking dish. Cover with a layer of lasagna noodles. Top with half the sliced meatballs, then sprinkle a few tablespoons of the mozzarella over them. Top with more lasagna noodles, add half the sliced meatballs, and sprinkle with 2 more tablespoons of the mozzarella. Top with remaining noodles. Top with remaining diced tomatoes and sprinkle with the remaining mozzarella. Bake 45 to 50 minutes, uncovered, until the cheese has melted and the edges are lightly browned. Let cool 5 minutes before cutting into eight squares and serving.

Nutritional Stats Per serving (serving size: 1 large [4-inch] slice of lasagna with meatballs) 343 calories, 23 g protein, 8 g sugars, 39 g carbohydrates, 11 g fat (5 g saturated), 50 mg cholesterol, 6 g fiber, 315 mg sodium

BAKED SHRIMP SCAMPI

Shrimp are high in dietary iodine, a superfood for your thyroid. Don't be concerned about the naturally occurring cholesterol found in shrimp and other shellfish like lobsters. Studies show that dietary cholesterol doesn't raise blood serum cholesterol.

Serves 4

1 pound medium peeled, deveined shrimp (about 22 per pound)
1 tablespoon olive oil
4 garlic cloves, minced
¼ teaspoon crushed red pepper flakes
⅛ teaspoon freshly grated black pepper
1 pound green beans, stems trimmed
¼ cup low-sodium chicken or vegetable broth
1 lemon plus additional lemon wedges, for serving
¼ cup minced fresh parsley leaves
6 ounces whole wheat or gluten-free spaghetti or angel hair pasta,
    cooked according to the package instructions

Preheat the oven to 400°F. Place the shrimp in a large bowl along with the olive oil, garlic, chili flakes, and black pepper, and toss well. Set aside.

Arrange the green beans in a 7 x 11-inch baking dish. Pour in the chicken broth. Layer the shrimp on top. Using a zester, zest the lemon over the top of the shrimp. Cover with aluminum foil and bake 25 minutes, until the shrimp are cooked through and no longer translucent and the beans are fork-tender. Serve immediately over the pasta.

Nutritional Stats Per serving (serving size: ¼ pound shrimp plus veggies and pasta) 306 calories, 25 g protein, 6 g sugars, 45 g carbohydrates, 5 g fat (1 g saturated), 143 mg cholesterol, 8 g fiber, 690 mg sodium

Chef's Note: This is a perfect entertaining dish that you can prep and refrigerate up to 4 hours before your guests arrive. Serve with whole-wheat store-bought garlic bread and leftover meatballs (page 338).

SALSA COD WITH GUACAMOLE

Storing avocado with its pit doesn't keep it from turning brown as was once thought. To keep overnight, place a layer of plastic wrap directly over the surface and store refrigerated, in an airtight container.

Serves 4

Salsa Cod
Four 4-ounce cod fillets
½ cup jarred salsa

Guacamole
2 large ripe avocados, preferably Hass
1 ripe tomato, seeded, finely chopped (about 1 cup)
¼ cup minced red onion
Juice of 2 limes (about ¼ cup)
1 jalapeño pepper, seeded and finely chopped (optional)
¼ cup minced fresh cilantro (optional)
¼ teaspoon sea salt

Preheat oven to 400°F. Place the fish in a 7 x 11-inch baking dish. Spread the salsa over the fish. Bake 15 to 18 minutes, until the fish flakes when pressed with a fork.

In the meanwhile make the guacamole. Place the avocados, tomato, onion, lime juice, jalapeño (if using), cilantro (if using), and salt in a large bowl. Use a wooden spoon to mash the ingredients together. Split into four even portions and serve immediately with the fish.

Nutritional Stats Per serving (serving size: 1 piece cod with ¼ cup guacamole) 327 calories, 26 g protein, 3 g sugars, 16 g carbohydrates, 20 g fat (3 g saturated), 57 mg cholesterol, 9 g fiber, 4087 mg sodium

BAKED COD WITH BASIL PESTO

"C" is for cauliflower since it has a surprisingly high vitamin C load, more than 70 percent of your daily needs in just one cup! So if you're looking for a super low-carb way to get more of this powerful detox nutrient, then cauliflower mash is your go-to side dish.

Serves 4

Cod
2 cups baby spinach
2 cups basil leaves
3 tablespoons olive oil
3 tablespoons walnuts
¼ salt
Four 4-ounce cod fillets

Cauliflower Mash
½ head cauliflower, cut into florets (about 4 cups)
1 tablespoon olive oil
2 teaspoon Dijon mustard
½ teaspoon chili powder
¼ teaspoon salt

Preheat oven to 400°F. To make the pesto, place the spinach, basil, olive oil, walnuts, and salt in a food processor. Process until a chunky mixture forms. Divide the pesto into four portions and spread over each piece of fish. Bake 18 to 20 minutes, until the fish flakes when pressed with a fork.

For the cauliflower mash, bring 1 inch of water to a boil in a large saucepan. Add the cauliflower and cover. Cook 4 to 5 minutes, until the cauliflower is fork-tender and most of the water has evaporated. Pour out any remaining water. Using a potato masher, fork, or food processor, mash until a chunky puree forms. Stir in the oil, mustard, chili powder, and salt, and serve immediately.

Nutritional Stats Per serving (serving size: 1 piece of pesto cod and 1 cup cauliflower mash) 302 calories, 27 g protein, 2 g sugars, 7 g carbohydrates, 19 g fat (3 g saturated), 57 mg cholesterol, 3 g fiber, 468 mg sodium

SLOW COOKER CHICKEN ENCHILADAS

Swapping canned beans for tortillas certainly brings down the sodium in this spin on chicken enchiladas while providing a wide array of heart-healthy nutrients, like folate and manganese (not to be confused with magnesium). Manganese helps your body regulate blood sugar and is important for glowing, healthy skin.

Serves 4

1 pound boneless, skinless chicken breasts (about 3 large or 4 small)
1 cup diced tomatoes
1 onion, diced
1 red bell pepper, seeded and diced
1 green bell pepper, seeded and diced
3 cloves garlic, minced
3 teaspoons paprika or chili powder, mild or hot
2 cups canned beans or cooked lentils

Place chicken, tomatoes, onion, red and green bell peppers, garlic, and paprika or chili powder in a slow cooker. Set on high and cook for 2½ hours, until the chicken is fork-tender. Remove the chicken and shred it. Return it to the cooker and add the beans or lentils. Let rest for 5 minutes to allow the beans or lentils to warm through. Spoon into four portions and serve immediately.

Nutritional Stats Per serving (serving size: about 1½ cups) 284 calories, 34 g protein, 11 g sugars, 27 g carbohydrates, 6 g fat (1 g saturated), 73 mg cholesterol, 8 g fiber, 635 mg sodium

If you feel that any of these dishes can use some "punching up," try some of these add-ons in moderation to fill the gaps.

CHEF ROCCO'S SEASONING SALT

Looking to give your meal more of an Italian spin? Add crushed fennel seeds and remove ginger for my Italian spice inspiration.

Makes 2 tablespoon seasoning salt

1 teaspoon no-salt-added garlic powder

1 teaspoon sea salt

1 teaspoon black peppercorns

1 teaspoon ground powdered ginger

1 teaspoon chili flakes

1 teaspoon lemon or lime zest

Place all ingredients in a spice grinder or clean coffee grinder and pulse about 30 seconds until a fine powder forms. Use immediately or store in an airtight container on the countertop until ready to use.

Nutritional Stats Per serving (¼ teaspoon) 1 calorie, 0 g protein, 0 g sugars, 0 g carbohydrates, 0 g fat (0 g saturated), 0 mg cholesterol, 0 g fiber, 98 mg sodium

Chef's Note: Seek out delicious sea salt—such as Maldon—that you can find in gourmet markets. Its flaky texture adds interest to your taste buds and makes cooking more fun!

SIMPLE SALT-FREE SUGAR-FREE BBQ SPICE

Use this to add a flavor punch to your favorite lean meats like chicken, fish, or flank steak. For a wet marinade, mix 1 tablespoon BBQ spice with 1 tablespoon olive oil.

Makes about 2 cups

½ cup lemon zest (from 4 lemons)

1 cup stevia

1 tablespoon cayenne

1 tablespoon salt-free garlic powder

1 tablespoon black pepper

½ teaspoon ground cumin

½ teaspoon dried cilantro or parsley

Place all ingredients in a spice grinder or clean coffee grinder and pulse about 30 seconds, until a fine powder forms. Use immediately or store in an airtight container on the countertop until ready to use.

Nutritional Stats Per serving (1 tablespoon) 3 calories, 0 g protein, 0 g sugars, 1 g carbohydrates, 0 g fat (0 g saturated), 0 mg cholesterol, 0 g fiber, 0 mg sodium

CHINESE FIVE SPICE

Use this guilt-free mixture on your Asian-inspired dishes, or anywhere you see fit.

Makes about ½ cup

1 tablespoon fennel seeds

5 to 6 star anise pods

1 tablespoon aniseed

1 tablespoon ground cinnamon

1 tablespoon black pepper

1 tablespoon ground clove

Place all ingredients in a spice grinder or clean coffee grinder and pulse about 30 seconds until a fine powder forms. Use immediately or store in an airtight container on the countertop until ready to use.

Nutritional Stats Per serving (¼ teaspoon) 2 calories, 0 g protein, 0 g sugars, 0 g carbohydrates, 0 g fat (0 g saturated), 0 mg cholesterol, 0 g fiber, 0 mg sodium

SALSA VERDE WITH CHIA SEEDS

This flavorful, rich-tasting salsa verde is easy to make with ingredients you'll already have in your pantry. For an amazing salad, combine 1 recipe of salsa verde with 4 cups baby kale. Cover and chill for 1 hour, then serve.

Makes ¼ cup

1 tablespoon chia seeds

2 tablespoons minced red onion

1 tablespoon vinegar, any type

1 tablespoon capers

1 tablespoon parsley

1 tablespoon olive oil

Place all the ingredients in a medium bowl. Toss well and chill at least 1 hour before serving.

Nutritional Stats Per serving (1 tablespoon) 53 calories, 0 g protein, 1 g sugars, 3 g carbohydrates, 4 g fat (0 g saturated), 0 mg cholesterol, 1 g fiber, 80 mg sodium

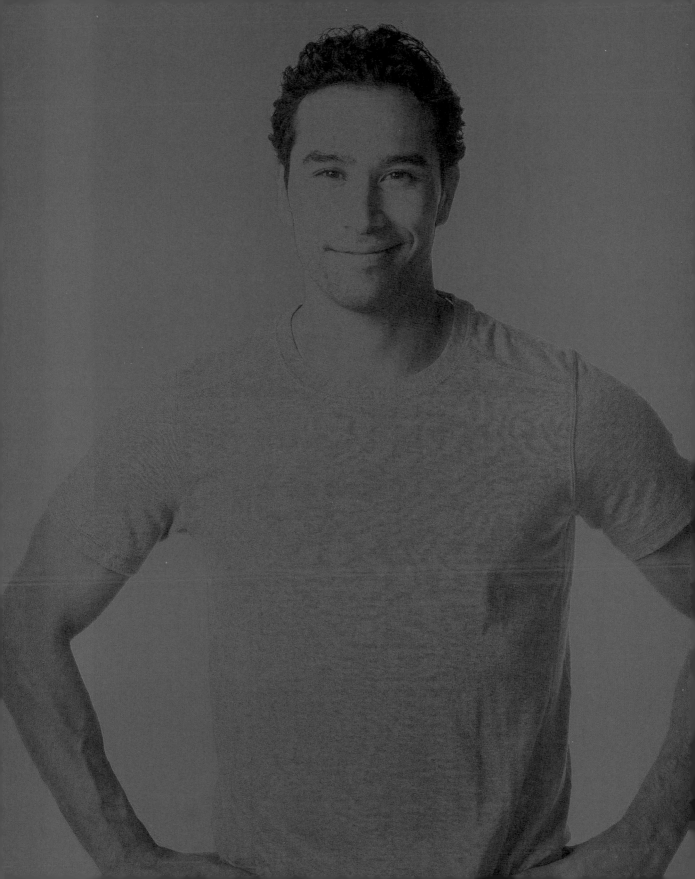

THIRTEEN

Sustain Your Results for Life

kai·zen (kahy-zen). noun.
1. A business philosophy or system that is based on making positive changes on a regular basis, as to improve productivity.
2. An approach to one's personal or social life that focuses on continuous improvement.

CONGRATULATIONS! YOU'VE DONE IT! You followed the *20-Minute Body* program to a T for 20 days and you have a lot of progress to show for it. But let's get serious for a moment. I'm telling you to save the high-fives for later, and focus on a big question: Where will you go from here? That's the question everyone has after finishing a regimented workout and nutrition program: Now what?

This chapter is all about the "now what." We're going to look at long-term personal change, and how you can take what you've learned and make it a part of your lifestyle.

KAIZEN: A FORCE FOR CONTINUOUS, POSITIVE CHANGE

My heritage is part Japanese and recently I had the opportunity to travel to Japan to train U.S. military personnel and meet members of my birth family. It was an incredibly moving trip for many reasons, and during that trip was introduced to the concept of *kaizen*, a philosophy of positive change in Japanese society. The term has been adapted to recognize the concept of constant improvement both in the business world and in our personal lives.

That's what I'm inviting you to do on day 21 of your program: commit to the idea that you're really at the beginning of a lifelong journey of continuous improvement. These first 20 days have given you a foundation for better health. The next step is to embrace the idea of *kaizen*—constant improvement—to set new goals and progress to even higher levels of achievement.

PROGRESS THROUGH THE COLOR LEVELS

You started at the yellow level. Depending on how challenging that 20-day cycle was for you, you might want to stay at the yellow level for another 20 days, adding in a few exercise progressions and nutrition variables. Or maybe you've mastered the yellow nutrition but not the workouts—so you want to stick with yellow workouts for another cycle, but go on to the orange meal plan. Or maybe you've mastered the whole thing and want to go straight to the orange level. Only you know the right next steps for you. You can customize the program in any way you'd like, as long as you don't skip levels.

And remember, no matter what the instructions for your workouts say, you can always make these exercises more challenging by adding resistance (exercise bands or hand weights), instability (standing on one leg, for example), or speed (trying to do more reps in the same amount of time). Review the material in Chapter 11 to create more challenging versions of these exercises.

SET NEW FITNESS GOALS

Now that you're feeling more fit, it's time to choose a new fitness goal. Choosing a new fitness goal is a great way to stay motivated and keep yourself accountable each step of the way. As you progress through the color levels, you should continually set new goals for yourself so that you have targets to hit, and can measure your success.

Maybe there's a new sport or activity that you've always wanted to try out. If so, now is the time! You're feeling fit and strong, and your confidence is soaring. Identify an activity you've always wanted to do and do an online search to find a beginners' group that meets near you. (Come to think of it, I live in Southern California and surfing sure looks like fun. *Hmm. . . .*)

Many of my clients start getting involved in fun road races like Tough Mudder, the Color Run, or the Rock and Roll series in their hometowns. If that's something that sounds like fun to you, stop in at a local running shoe store to see if it has group workouts (almost every store does). Find a group that's at your level to start with, and go for it!

And if you do decide to train for an athletic event, you can still do another 20-day cycle of this program. Taking 20 minutes a day to do these exercises will help give you the strength, stamina, and flexibility for any physical challenge you want to conquer.

BUT THERE'S MORE

One 20-day cycle of my program is like a honeymoon. Admittedly, it's a pretty athletic honeymoon! But the excitement and commitment are all

DINING OUT

Sure, you were laser-focused on your nutrition for 20 days, but now what? Life doesn't occur in a vacuum. Every once in a while you need to eat out. Whether you have friends or family to entertain, your boss is taking the team out to a dinner, or you just need a change of scenery, going out can be every bit as enjoyable and productive for your mind *and* body as eating at home. Here are some tips to help you make sure you don't stray too far from your healthy eating plan:

· If you're meeting friends for dinner, don't arrive early and wait for them at the bar. That's temptation overload. Arrive a bit later than your friends and go right to your table.

· Start your meal with a vegetable-based soup or a salad with a simple dressing of olive oil and lemon juice or vinegar.

· Ask the server to take away the bread basket.

· Scope out the restaurant before you arrive. Just about every restaurant now has an online menu. Decide in advance what you'd like to order.

· Order sauces and dressings on the side and dip your fork in them to get the taste of the sauce without all of the calories.

· Order a healthy appetizer and split a main course with a friend.

· Eat slowly. Savor every bite. Enjoy the company of your friends as well as the meal.

· In the real world outside your kitchen, you can't control every ingredient—but that's the point of dining out. Enjoy new foods, appreciate a chef's skills, and stick to your routine as best you can. Finding pleasure and flavor in wholesome, delicious food is a healthy part of your new life.

there and it's only 20 days, so chances are you didn't lose focus on the program during this time. But *fitness from within* isn't a honeymoon—it's a marriage. It's much easier to carve out the time to commit to a short program than it is to figure out how to make life changes that are going to last for the long haul, but that's exactly what I'm asking you to do . . . for you, and for the "why" you committed to early on.

Remember my history of being overweight as a teenager? When I started to change my life, I embraced new challenges, especially martial arts. As I progressed and started to feel my body changing, I knew I wanted to feel healthy all the time. I committed myself to long-term changes, even when I wanted to go back to old habits. And the easiest way to create a new habit is to replace an old habit with a better one. Instead of wandering to the food pantry when I was bored, I would practice a new karate routine, or something similar. That would "wake up" my brain—the part of me that had an old, ingrained habit just waiting there to be woken up when I was bored or upset again. And instead of just blindly going to the pantry, I'd be able to say to myself, *Brett, you know where this leads. Do something positive instead.*

Whether you call it willpower or commitment or use another term, here's the deal: it's a muscle. Just like your physical muscles, your mental muscles get strengthened every time you resist doing something you know isn't good for you, and instead choose a healthier option. The more you do it, the easier it gets.

So, how do you keep a muscle strong? Two ways, really. First, you use it often enough that it gets challenged, so that it adapts to the new demands being put on it. And second, you try not to pre-fatigue it with doubt before asking it to be strong for you.

DON'T PRE-FATIGUE YOUR MENTAL MUSCLES!

If I'm doing a *20-Minute Body* workout, I want to start fresh and well rested. If, before I start the workout, I do something physically challenging like carrying a huge bag of groceries up a staircase, I'll take the time to rest for a few minutes before starting my workout, in order to let my heart return to a rest state and let my muscles relax.

If I don't do this, my muscles will already be tired when the workout begins, and I won't get as much value from the workout because my muscles won't be able to perform at the high level I'm asking of them.

Our mental muscles work in exactly the same way.

If you want to succeed in making fitness a lifestyle, you need to prioritize the things that make it possible: time for your workouts, healthy meals, and mental training. A great way to do that is to work out first thing in the morning, shop for groceries on the weekends, and prepare meals as much in advance as you can.

Let's say you push your workout to the evening. Who knows what might happen during the day that could pre-fatigue your mental muscles to the point where you not only skip your daily workout, but end up at the doughnut shop on the corner? If you work a stressful 12-hour workday, have a tense conversation with your boss, and then come home and have a fight with your partner because you're so tired and stressed, what's going to happen next? Pizza? Wine? Chips? More often than not, you'll fall back into old, unhealthy routines, because your mental muscles are just plain tired.

When I see ads for "low calorie" processed treats I worry that people use them too often as a crutch. In the situation that I described above, is a low-calorie doughnut (which is probably full of chemicals and artificial sweeteners) going to make anything in your life better? Isn't that just a Band-Aid attempting to fix a much deeper problem? The solution to any stressor or problem isn't to grab a treat (and good luck eating just one, by the way). The solution is to realize what happened when you chose not to prioritize your health. You asked too much of your mental muscles, so that by the end of the day you threw up your hands in defeat.

Strengthen your mental muscles by prioritizing your health and fitness every day. Just like lifting a heavier weight, it gets easier with practice.

GOING FURTHER: HOW TO CREATE YOUR OWN WORKOUTS

The 4x4, Double Trouble, Triple Threat, 30 HI–30 LO, and 100s workouts provide not only specific exercises to keep you challenged, but also a framework for how to make up your own workouts. This has two benefits: you'll keep yourself constantly challenged, and you'll start to take ownership of your health by making decisions about what exercises and workouts are best for you over time.

For example, let's look a little closer at the 4x4. Here's the basic structure of the 4x4 workout:

- It's made up of four exercises (one each for upper body, lower body, cardio, and abs/core).

- Each exercise is performed for 1 minute

- All four exercises are performed in a row (for 4 minutes total).

- You rest for 1 minute between the 4-minute sets.

- You repeat the entire 4-minute set with 1 minute of rest four times total for a 20-minute workout

That's all it is. So, how can you create your own 4x4 workout? Let's say you're on the road and you need to get in a workout, and you happened to bring your exercise band with you. What might your own 4x4 look like? Here's just one idea:

- **EXERCISE 1. SHOULDERS:** Shoulder raises with exercise band (page 145)

- **EXERCISE 2. BACK:** One-leg deadlift with row (with band) (Page 147)

- **EXERCISE 3. LEGS AND UPPER BODY:** Thrusters (squat + overhead press) (page 178)

- **EXERCISE 4. ABS AND CORE:** Crossover plank with Spiderman kick (page 162)

And there you go. It really is that simple. Over time, you'll find that you can create your own workouts using the basic guidelines you've learned here. Be creative, try new movements, and above all, have fun!

"OUT OF THE BOX" GOALS

I like to say that fitness gave me my freedom. When I finally took stock of my own life and decided that I was going to be accountable to my word, everything changed. Fitness is more than a great pair of jeans, a six-pack, or a sexy swimsuit. It's a way for you to find out what you're made of and to apply that determination, knowledge, and energy to all of your life goals.

During your mental exercises, I asked you to start thinking about "out of the box" goals. Now is the time to really dedicate yourself to figuring out what those goals might be for you. "Out of the box" goals are the goals that aren't necessarily related to losing weight or getting fit. They can be much more expansive. They make you dream. They make you excited and hopeful for the future. What have you always dreamed of doing? Figure out what it is and go get it.

You might just find that the increased confidence you now have as a result of the discipline and focus you've brought to your *20-Minute Body* program propels you to new heights. Whatever you do, make it something really special—a reach goal, something that's a big jump for you right now—and then treat it just like this program. Take small, specific steps, track your progress, look for experts to help you along the way, and never give up!

Thanks for being with me on this journey. I wrote this book with my clients past, present, and future—people just like you—in my mind and heart. In the end, you did more than just give me or the program 20 days of your time . . . you gave your family, your body, and most of all yourself a priceless gift. What will you do with the next 20 days? Time to go find out. . . .

Acknowledgments

THIS BOOK is part of a continual process of learning and growing in all aspects of life. I knew I wanted to put my ideas to paper, but two friends helped set things in motion to make it come to fruition. The first is *New York Times* bestselling author JJ Virgin, who I met while filming the Food Network show *Fat Chef*. She introduced me to her literary agent, Celeste Fine, who became my agent and really got things rolling. The second friend who helped make this book a reality is Nicole Dunn of Dunn Pellier Media, who introduced me to my publisher soon after I told her I was moving forward with my book. Without their belief in me and willingness to help, I may not have written it.

I am so grateful to the many people who have helped inspire me to develop the passion, knowledge, and programs reflected in these pages. To list everyone by name would take up more than half the book, but I would like to single out the following:

To my mother and father, for giving the love and support that's been the pillar of strength in my life. You adopted me and raised me with unconditional love. You led by example, and I hope I am a living proof of all that you taught me and all that you represent. I miss you both more than you know. To my extended family for teaching me so many valuable lessons, being such inspirational role models, and helping shape me into the person I am today.

To my birth mother, for having the courage and trust to place me for adoption and for making our reunion more meaningful than I ever could have imagined. I love you.

To Celeste Fine, thank you for seeing and believing in my vision and going above and beyond the call of an agent.

To Julie Will, editor at Harper Collins, and her staff, for immediately resonating with my ideas and helping craft the book into what it is today.

To Eric Velazquez, you picked the project up at the one yard line and carried it home.

To Chef Rocco Whalen and Chef Jennifer Iserloh for their friendship and incredible skill and knowledge to make the recipes in the book truly incredible.

To my team at Hoebel Fitness for all their long hours and unwavering support, which allowed me to write this book with all the many other things going on in my life.

To the trainers and staff at Peak Performance Gym in New York City, you have inspired and pushed me to always strive to be better. Knowledge is power, but applied knowledge is priceless.

To Jillian Michaels, Bob Harper, Cara Castronuova, and the contestants on *The Biggest Loser*, the experience with you all changed my life, and I will always be grateful.

To Carl Daikeler, Lara Ross, and the Beachbody team, for giving me an amazing opportunity to work with you and learn from the best. You believed in me and my program and showed tremendous tenacity.

You all have inspired and changed me in many ways. Words are not enough, but the one quote that comes to mind is by Sir Isaac Newton:

"If I have seen further, it is by standing on the shoulders of giants."

Much love,
Brett

Notes

[1] Tremblay, A., J. Simoneau, and C. Bouchard. "Impact of exercise intensity on body fatness and skeletal muscle metabolism." *Metabolism*, July 1994. http://www.ncbi.nlm.nih.gov/pubmed/8028502.

[2] Jensen, L., J. Bangsbo, and Y. Hellsten. "Effect of high intensity training on capillarization and presence of angiogenic factors in human skeletal muscle." *Journal of Physiology,* March 2004: 557, 571–82. http://jp.physoc.org/content/557/2/571.

[3] Westcott, W. "Increased muscle = increased resting metabolic rates = weight loss." http://bit .ly/1tKfLMK.

[4] Bollinger, L., and T. LaFontaine. "Exercise and insulin resistance." *Strength and Conditioning Journal*, July 2011.

[5] Black, L., P. Swan, and B. Alvar. "Effects of intensity and volume on insulin sensitivity during acute bouts of resistance training." *Journal of Strength and Conditioning* 24(4) 2010: 1109–16.

[6] Dukette, Dianne, and David Cornish. *The Essential 20: Twenty Components of an Excellent Health Care Team* (Pittsburgh: RoseDog Books, 2009), 72–73.

[7] Flood-Obbagy, J., and B. Rolls. "The effect of fruit in different forms on energy intake and satiety at a meal." *Appetite,* April 2009. www.ncbi.nlm.nih.gov/pmc/articles/PMC2664987/.

[8] Duhigg, Charles. *The Power of Habit: Why We Do What We Do in Life and Business* (NY: Random House, 2012).

[9] Macpherson, R., T. Hazell, T. Olver, et al. "Run sprint interval training improves aerobic performance but not maximal cardiac output." *Medicine & Science in Sports & Exercise*, January 2011. http://www.ncbi.nlm.nih.gov/pubmed/20473222.

[10] Tremblay et al. "Impact of exercise intensity on body fatness and skeletal muscle metabolism."

[11] King, J. "A comparison of the effects of interval training vs. continuous training on weight loss and body composition in obese pre-menopausal women." *Electronic Theses and Dissertations,* Paper 123, 2001. http://dc.etsu.edu/etd/123.

[12] Trapp, E., D. Chisholm, J. Freund, et al. "The effects of high-intensity intermittent exercise training on fat loss and fasting insulin levels of young women." *International Journal of Obesity,* April 2008.

[13] Stokes, K., M. Nevill, G. Hall, et al. "The time course of the human growth hormone response to a 6 s and a 30 s cycle ergometer sprint." *Journal of Sports Sciences,* June 2002.

[14] Dolezal, B., J. Potteiger, and D. Jacobsen. "Muscle damage and resting metabolic rate after acute resistance exercise with an eccentric overload." *Medicine & Science in Sports & Exercise,* July 2000.

[15] Ratamess, N., M. Falvo, G. Mangine, et al. "The effect of rest interval length on metabolic responses to the bench press exercise." *European Journal of Applied Physiology,* May 2007.

[16] American Physiological Society. "Minutes of hard exercise can lead to all-day calorie burn." www.eurekalert.org/pub_releases/2012-10/aps-moh101112.php.

[17] Ibid.

[18] Stokes et al., "The time course of the human growth hormone response to a 6 s and a 30 s cycle ergometer sprint."

[19] "Nursing your sweet tooth." www.forbes.com/sites/alicegwalton/2012/08/30/how-much-sugar-are-americans-eating-infographic/.

[20] Thompson, D. "Four foods to avoid that promote inflammation and can cause disease." http://blogs.kqed.org/bayareabites/2013/02/20/four-foods-to-avoid-that-promote-inflammation-and-can-cause-disease/.

[21] Yang, Q., Z. Zhang, E. Gregg, et al. "Added sugar intake and cardiovascular diseases mortality among US adults." *JAMA Internal Medicine,* April 2014.

[22] Mayo Clinic. "Artificial sweeteners and other sugar substitutes." www.mayoclinic.org/healthy-living/nutrition-and-healthy-eating/in-depth/artificial-sweeteners/art-20046936?pg=1.

[23] Harvard Health Publications. "Artificial sweeteners: Sugar-free, but at what cost?" www.health.harvard.edu/blog/artificial-sweeteners-sugar-free-but-at-what-cost-201207165030.

[24] He, F., C. Nowson, M. Lucas, et al. "Increased consumption of fruit and vegetables is related to a reduced risk of coronary heart disease: Meta-analysis of cohort studies." *Journal of Human Hypertension,* 2007.

[25] Egner, P., J. Chen, A. Zarth, et al. "Rapid and sustainable detoxification of airborne pollutants by broccoli sprout beverage: Results of a randomized clinical trial in China." *Cancer Prevention Research*, June 2014.

[26] Centers for Disease Control and Prevention. "What does moderate drinking mean?" www.cdc.gov/alcohol/faqs.htm#moderateDrinking.

[27] Mayo Clinic. "Red wine and resveratrol: Good for your heart?" www.mayoclinic.org/diseases-conditions/heart-disease/in-depth/red-wine/art-20048281.

[28] "Mai tai nutrition." http://caloriecount.about.com/calories-mai-tai-ic1413.

[29] "Calories in wine, table, red." http://caloriecount.about.com/calories-wine-table-red-i14096.

[30] "Sleep curtailment in healthy young men is associated with decreased leptin levels, elevated ghrelin levels, and increased hunger and appetite." http://isites.harvard.edu/fs/docs/icb.topic197607.files/Due_Wk_11_Nov_28/SPIEGEL_2004.pdf.

[31] Source: www.whfoods.com/genpage.php?tname=nutrient&ibid=77.

[32] Source: www.ncbi.nlm.nih.gov/pubmed/23225499.

[33] Source: www.naturalnews.com/042568_plant_hormones_broccoli_cancer-fighting_potential.html.

About the Author

Founder of Hoebel Fitness, Brett Hoebel is a fitness expert and former trainer on *The Biggest Loser*. A 15-year veteran in the fitness industry, Brett has shaped-up Hollywood's finest, including Victoria's Secret supermodels and A-list actors. He appears frequently on shows like *The Dr. Oz Show*, *The Talk*, *The View*, and *Today*, and is a contributing fitness expert for publications including *Fitness*, *Self*, *Women's Health*, *Vogue*, and *Details*.

Find him online at bretthoebel.com, and connect with him on social media at facebook.com/bretthoebel and @bretthoebel.